MW01620387

# Whispers from the East

Applying the Principles of Eastern Healing to Psychotherapy

# Whispers from the East

Frances E. Steinberg, Ph.D.,
and Richard G. Whiteside, M.S.W.

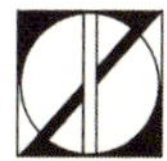

Zeig, Tucker & Co., Inc., Publishers
Phoenix, Arizona

Published by
Zeig, Tucker & Co., Inc.
1928 East Highland, Suite F104-607
Phoenix, Arizona 85020

Library of Congress Cataloging–in–Publication Data

Steinberg, Frances E., 1951–
Whispers from the East : applying the principles of eastern healing to psychotherapy / Frances E. Steinberg and Richard G. Whiteside.
p. cm.
Includes bibliographical references and index.
ISBN 1-891944-04-5
1. Psychotherapy. 2. Medicine, Chinese. 3. Mind and body therapies. I. Whiteside, Richard G. II. Title.
RC480.5.S675 1998
616.89'14—dc21 98-38991
CIP

Manufactured in the United States of America
10 9 8 7 6 5 4 3 2 1

■

In memory of Harriet Scharogrodsky Steinberg,
who had enough room on her lap to rock the whole world.

# ACKNOWLEDGMENTS

This book actually began in a traffic jam on the Baltimore Beltway in 1993. Sitting there in frustration, the authors, in an attempt to maintain sanity, began to discuss what they felt would be the next major shift in philosophy in family therapy. Rick Whiteside maintained that for decades all of the new models had been first-order changes and that the field was primed for a radical second-order adjustment. Frances Steinberg said that perhaps what was needed was an entirely new way of looking at things, and she pointed to the Eastern healing Law of Five Elements. Then the traffic started to move, and the conversation and car shifted to other things and places. Over the next few years, however, the ideas begun in the snarl began to reappear in enough other contexts that the authors decided it was time to do something about them.

The authors owe thanks to a variety of sources involved with the formulation and completion of the project. Rick is indebted to the *yin* and *yang* of his training, Cloe Madanes and Jay Haley, who introduced him to Eastern philosophy in the context of family therapy. Frances would like to thank all of her acupuncture teachers, particularly J. Michael Moore and Stuart Watts, for the wealth of information they shared and their patience in showing a confirmed empiricist the "way." The authors are also indebted to Zeig, Tucker & Co. for having the courage to support such a nontraditional project, with a special "thank you" to editor Suzi Tucker, who applies both sharpened pencil and insight with tremendous care.

# CONTENTS

■

# Whispers from the East

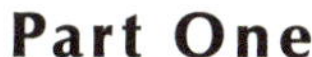

# Part One

## INTRODUCTION

*The ancient masters were subtle, mysterious,*
*profound, responsive.*
*The depth of their knowledge is unfathomable.*

*—Lao-tzu*

In the current climate of managed care, accountability, and financial crunches, it is sometimes difficult to remember that therapy is essentially a healing profession. A desire to fill in insurance forms, track client hours, or establish performance criteria was not why most therapists entered the field. A more likely motivation was a desire to help and to facilitate well-being in others, a goal that can be lost in the overwhelming, daily details of practice.

In this book, principles of Eastern (or Oriental) healing are woven into the practice of modern psychotherapy in an effort to rekindle the therapist's healing drive. Many of the concepts in the fields of acupuncture and herbology are thousands of years old and so carry the force of a million healings. More important, the timeless wisdom they encompass allows us to step back from the limitations of our daily lives and view ourselves and our clients from a broader perspective. The book is not intended as a "how to," but as more of a spiritual tickle, an understanding that sits to the left of awareness.

■

## The Web

A fundamental lesson of Eastern healing is that everything is connected. A holistic approach has always characterized Chinese medicine, with no one part of the body considered separable from any other. As a logical corollary, since all things are related, changing any one of them should create a shift in the others. In acupuncture, for instance, because all of the channels of energy flow and physiological organs connect on a variety of levels, stimulating a point on one meridian can resolve a problem on another. Obviously, some choices of treatment are more sensible than others. One would not necessarily go to London from New York via Beijing, but it is possible.

The same thing is true if one adopts this attitude with regard to therapy. Systems of connections are present on both intrapersonal and interpersonal levels, so that creating a shift at any point can produce concomitant transformations at another. Both psychodynamic and family systems therapy acknowledge this web of relatedness. Within a therapeutic context, for instance, when presented with an identified patient who is a delinquent teenager, one might choose to work individually with the youngster, intervene with the parents, or add a community youth worker to the mix. Depending on the selection, changes will be sudden or slow, temporary or long term, significant or trivial. What often makes a difference is whether sufficient energy has been invested in the process to produce a significant alteration of the circumstances. Most intrapersonal and interpersonal systems tend toward inertia. In order for therapy to be successful, there must be enough impetus to move the balance point so that a new homeostatic level can be found.

In Eastern medicine, there also is no differentiation between emotional and physical symptoms—both are expected and accepted in every case. Bloodshot eyes, a migraine headache, and explosive anger are regarded as equally important manifestations of the same condition—liver fire rising. There is no attempt either to elevate or to denigrate the value of physical or emotional components. They are not two sides of the same coin; they are both elements of the metals that make up that coin.

It is not always viewed that way in therapy. Consider Tommy, a 16-year-old who experienced blackouts while running. He often couldn't remember sequences of time; he only knew he had been in one place and then in another. The doctors suspected epilepsy or a brain tumor, but neurological assessments revealed nothing unusual. He was then sent to a series of psychiatrists, who eventually diagnosed Tommy as having a dissociative disorder. The most interesting feature of the case was how differently the professionals and the family reacted after Tommy had received a psychiatric label as compared with their reactions when Tommy's problem was thought to be neurological. As a patient with a medical disorder, Tommy commanded a high level of concern, but as one with a psychiatric syndrome, he was considered defective in some way. At the heart of the matter, however, is the fact that his symptoms didn't change, but only the framing of them did.

The interrelationship of emotions and physical well-being has attracted increasing attention on the part of both therapy and medicine in recent years. It is now commonly accepted, for instance, that through meditation or imagery techniques, one can affect certain somatic ailments and assist healing. Similarly, it is currently believed that medical conditions, including such discrete events as heart surgery, produce specific emotional reactions in many patients. In both of these situations, however, the physical body and its mental/emotional/spiritual aspects are still viewed as separate. It is acknowledged that they influence each other, interacting in positive and negative ways to cause either healing or disease, but they are regarded as conceptually different in their makeup.

Eastern medicine pushes us further and asks whether it ever makes sense to consider the body and the psyche as discrete or separate. It also begs us to consider why we generally regard illnesses of the body as more "real" and of greater value than mental problems, so that patients with problems of psychogenic origin or manifestation are held in lower esteem than those whose diseases are believed to be somatic.

Traditionally, in Chinese medicine, the seven emotions—anger, joy, grief, melancholy, worry, fear, and fright—have been considered the primary causes of internal disease. Unusually severe or prolonged exposure to any of them would produce radical changes in a person's health and significantly affect one's *qi* ("chee"), or energy. With anger, energy rises in the body, resulting in such complaints as migraines and vertigo, while fear makes energy sink, causing such symptoms as enuresis. Excessive joy induces the *qi* to move more slowly (contentment breeding complacency and lack of growth), and worry causes it to stagnate even further, keeping people stuck in their problems and creating such conditions as arthritis or tumors. Both grief and melancholy consume energy, weakening both body and spirit, and fright often causes *qi* to become "deranged," scattering it in every direction and so producing irrational behavior. These classical descriptions of emotional consequences, however, are not as significant as is their lack of pejorative content. In the Eastern medical system, a person is not considered defective or inadequate if stress or trauma has caused a physical or behavioral symptom; indeed, it is expected.

## ANTIPATHOGENIC *QI*

Of equal importance is the explanation of why emotional events have significant effects at some times and not at others, a situation related to a factor called antipathogenic *qi*. Antipathogenic *qi* can be likened to the immune system, in that its primary function in Chinese medicine is to keep the body safe from harmful external influences. If the antipathogenic *qi* is high, a person can withstand significant trauma; if it is low, the slightest hiccup creates distress. Acupuncture treatment is generally directed toward improving the level of antipathogenic *qi*, since this enables one to handle life's ups and downs with less consequence.

Antipathogenic *qi* is comparable to the medical/psychological concept of diathesis, the predisposition of a body to disease. A person's diathesis comprises every factor and event that has occurred, both biologically and experientially, up to a particular time. All genetic, organic, cultural, familial, social, and educational experiences combine to make an individual unique to that moment, since each allele, trauma, and casual glance that the person has experienced helps to create the final product. It is onto this diathetic template that the world throws its stressors. If the diathesis is strong, it can absorb or handle significant crises. If the diathesis is weak, even breaking a fingernail can be a momentous event. This explains why some individuals have the capacity for resilience even in the face of shattering experiences whereas others need help in coping with daily stress.

According to traditional Chinese medicine, disease can occur when:

1. The level of antipathogenic *qi* is good, but the environmental event is so severe, prolonged, or unexpected that the body cannot defend against it.
2. Or the level of antipathogenic *qi* is so low that minimal environmental events have a significant impact.

In the first circumstance, individuals with a strong diathesis can become overwhelmed when a life event is so powerful that their normal means of coping are inadequate.

Nine-year-old Craig had handled the divorce of his parents fairly well. He missed the daily contact with Brian, his father, but enjoyed a good relationship with his mother, Sarah, and his six-year-old sister, Amy. Craig was able to see his father on most weekends, and although he preferred the comfort of his own bed to sleeping on his dad's couch, he loved the sloppier, more relaxed atmosphere of his father's apartment.

One night, Craig heard his mother arguing with his father on the telephone. At first, he didn't think anything was unusual since their frequent fighting had been the main reason for their separation, but after hanging up the phone, his mother went into the den and started crying. Craig tried to comfort her, but she assured him that she was all right, and he went to his room to watch TV. A short time later, Craig heard screaming from the den, and then the smoke alarm went off. As he ran downstairs, he saw his father leave through the front door. Craig called to him, but his father ignored him and jumped into his car. When Craig reached the den, he saw his mother in flames. He pushed her to the floor and wrapped her in a rug, as he had seen someone do on TV. When Amy came into the room and started crying, Craig told her to call 911 and ask for an ambulance.

The next several months were very difficult for Craig. He and Amy stayed with their grandmother while their mother recovered in the hospital. Brian was arrested for pouring gasoline over Sarah and intentionally setting her afire. Craig found it difficult to eat or sleep and began to wet his bed. He engaged in inappropriate actions at school, such as stealing from other children's desks and refusing to do his work.

Craig was strong enough to withstand the turmoil of his parents' disharmony and subsequent divorce. But when the intensity of the events accelerated to an extreme level, his ability to cope vanished, resulting in deteriorating behavior.

A similar effect can be produced by life events that may not be dramatic, but persist over time. For example, an intelligent, attractive woman who is continually belittled by her spouse may come to doubt her own self-worth. In the same way, individuals who spend extended time in institutions may progressively lose their ability to cope in the real world. In addition to stresses that are extreme or prolonged, events that are unexpected, such as the sudden loss of employment or the untimely death of a relative, can cause a normally competent person to experience difficulties in functioning.

Individuals with weak antipathogenic *qi* perceive minor events as challenging, and they have little protection from daily stress.

> Lena had raised her 12-year-old son, Peter, by herself since her husband had left the family when Peter was a baby. She worked as a bookkeeper, but often her income was insufficient to meet the bills. Lena ended each day feeling exhausted and overburdened. Her mother was critical of the way she parented Peter, and complained that none of the men her daughter met were good enough for her. As a result, Lena rarely dated. The family presented for therapy because Lena felt she could not control Peter. She described herself as a nag and Peter as difficult. When asked what the boy did that prompted her to correct him, she described such things as overeating at dinner and wanting to go to a friend's house to play.

Peter's behavior was not overly difficult or extreme, but it was too much for Lena to cope with because her antipathogenic *qi* was depleted. Within the conceptualization of Eastern medicine, there is a continual interplay between the underlying issues, in the form of antipathogenic *qi*, and the presenting context. In psychotherapy, therapists often choose to focus on either the causative or controlling issues of a problem, depending on their theoretical orientation. From the Eastern medical perspective, although it is often easiest to change the stressors, this must be done in the context of the individual's diathesis, since the ultimate goal is to strengthen the quality of the antipathogenic *qi* to ensure that health and balance can be maintained over the long run.

One of the most significant aspects of Eastern healing is the concept of intent, one's state of mind at the time of an action. Acupuncturists are taught to envision the flow of energy they wish to restore, focusing on the purpose of a needle as they insert it. This allows the practitioner's intent to penetrate the skin along with the needle.

Intensity of focus accomplishes several goals. First, the practitioner's technique is transformed from a routine procedure to a significant event. All of the practitioner's attention is focused on the act, making it an occasion of importance. This enables each insertion to acquire status, and its relationship to the system as a whole is reinforced. The acupuncture classics stress the significance of such focus by imploring practitioners to hold a needle as if they were grasping a tiger by its tail, a visualization that encourages the acupuncturist to be both careful and attentive. Poor choices of treatment can often be compensated for by purity of motive.

Analogously, in psychotherapy, there also should be intensive focus on each detail of the therapeutic exchange. Unfortunately, over the years, or even in the course of a day, as experience increases and boredom grows, the significance of each encounter with a client seems to lessen. In order to give each client the attention he or she deserves, therapists need to find ways of narrowing their focus so that intensity remains high. Samurai traditionally achieved this by visualizing themselves as living each moment as if their hair were on fire. In actuality, any means of bringing one back to the moment can work, whether it's performing a ritual before each client or having a colleague observe your therapy.

It must be considered, however, that our intent as practitioners isn't always perceived by our clients in the same way. One acupuncturist, for example, would sit quietly for a moment before treating a patient, placing his hands together and concentrating on gathering his energy before he took the person's pulse. The action reminded him to put all of his other issues aside and focus on the healing at hand. One day, as he put his hands together, the patient said, "I hope that things aren't so bad that you need to pray for me."

Intent also facilitates the achievement of specific goals in the healing context. In one system of acupuncture, rotating a needle clockwise once it is inserted is felt to increase the amount of energy in the needle's point. In another system, rotating the needle counterclockwise is assumed to produce the same result. Obviously, on an intellectual level, the systems can't both be correct, although they are equally successful. It is the practitioner's intention that produces the effect, not the technique. Therapists also benefit from having a clear concept as to the direction a particular session should take. Intent helps to focus their therapy, propelling their work toward success even when inadequate methods are used.

There are numerous approaches in psychotherapy that seem to achieve results almost in spite of the procedures used. It is often the therapist's belief in what he or she is doing, his or her intent, and the client's trust in the therapist, that achieves the therapeutic goals. This is congruent with the fact that the way that many therapists describe their work often differs greatly from what they actually do. The outcome of the therapy is usually linked to their intent, rather than to their actual practice.

Master-level therapists may possess enormous levels of intent, often to the point where they can achieve success with a technique that would fail miserably if used by a less dynamic therapist. Cloe Madanes, for instance, has written extensively on the importance of putting parents hierarchically in charge of their children on both a nurturing and a power level (Madanes, 1981). Madanes possesses the intent and charisma, however, to reverse this position when the need arises. For instance, she is able to invert the hierarchy, putting the children in charge of the parents to overcome a problem the parents are having (Madanes, 1984). Madanes maintains a clear sense of how to attain the goal of the therapy, using both her intent and her logic to detail the steps necessary to carry it through. When a novice therapist attempted a similar intervention with a family, but without the force of intent to execute the approach properly, the parents expressed anger that the therapist was siding with the children against them, and the children emerged as unruly tyrants.

Still, at times, it is the beginning therapist who possesses the power of intent. Therapists often start out as enthusiastic disciples of a particular method. Whether they are designing interventions, crafting letters, co-creating realities, or tapping on a client's wrist, their belief in the effectiveness of their technique means that it has a better chance of succeeding. Problems usually occur when the procedure becomes routine and stale. Then, therapists need to wake up their focus—to take a seminar, try a new strategy, read a book, in short, to do anything that will help them to bring the magic of intent back into their practice. We owe it to our clients to bring that focus and creativity into all of our interactions with them.

# CHAPTER ONE

## Fundamentals of Eastern Medicine

■

*The Tao begot one.*
*One begot two.*
*Two begot three.*
*And three begot the ten thousand things*
*—Lao-tzu*

The physiology of Eastern medicine is very different from that of the West. Here, organs are functional rather than anatomical, and the body contains patterns and substances that are not listed in any Western medical textbook. In order to understand the Eastern healing arts, one must first grasp the basics.

### THE BUILDING BLOCKS

#### *Qi*

*Qi* ("chee") is most commonly defined as "energy," but that is really an oversimplification; in the Eastern medical system, *qi* is actually the fundamental substance constituting the universe. It is energy at the point of materialization; matter at the point of energizing. It is the vital component of every person and object on the planet. *Qi* makes things happen and helps things live.

Each person actually possesses several types of *qi*. *Yuan* ("you-ahn") *qi*, inherited or source *qi*, comes from one's parents. It is the power source of the body, the core generator, the basis for and catalyst of all activity. The kernel of source *qi* inherited from one's parents can be conserved or used, but never replaced, so a concerted effort must be made to preserve it intact by using other sorts of *qi* for daily consumption. Source *qi* is analogous to the principal in a monetary investment—you can spend it if you have to, but it would be better to live off the interest.

It is preferable, then, to use *qi* that is obtained from acquired sources. The air that we breathe and the food we consume both bring *qi* into the body. Obviously, the caliber of what is ingested has a lot to do with the quantity and quality of the *qi* produced. The computer phrase "garbage in, garbage out" is highly applicable to *qi* production. If you breathe polluted air and eat junk food, you will not have much quality energy to use. If your intake is sufficiently depleted, the level of acquired *qi* will be so low that you will have to start using your *yuan qi* for daily functioning, which can have serious consequences.

Robin, a 14-year-old anorexic, was admitted to the hospital. At five feet, seven inches tall, she weighed only 65 pounds. Robin refused to ingest any food orally. She was so weak that it was an effort for her to talk, and she could not sit up in bed. Intravenous feeding was having little effect, and gradually Robin's physiological systems began to fail.

Robin's persistent lack of food intake had resulted in such a deficit of acquired *qi* that she needed to consume her *yuan qi* in order to function. Her core processes were so disrupted that Robin was unable to utilize the nourishment that was being supplied intravenously, and her organs began to fail.

Acquired *qi* moves through the body in a constant, repetitive pattern. Meridians (the channels through which the energy flows) are found both deep within and on the surface of the body, and bring *qi* to the organs, the limbs, and the skin, ensuring their proper functioning. This *qi* presents at various points on the surface of the body that are used by acupuncturists during treatment. By pressing on these spots or inserting a needle into them, an acupuncturist can access the flow of energy and restore health to the interior of the body. Developments in bioelectrical photography and histological structure analysis have confirmed the existence of the points that were identified experientially thousands of years ago (Hou, 1979; Plummer, 1980).

*Qi* serves five major functions in the body.

1. *It is the source of all movement in the body and accompanies all movement.* *Qi* is responsible for things happening at every level. No change, growth, or processing is possible without sufficient *qi*. Depression or an inability to change could be related to an insufficiency of *qi*. Healthy functioning occurs when *qi* is allowed to flow smoothly and without obstruction. Problems on both an intrapersonal and an interpersonal level occur when *qi* flow is impaired. Obsession with the past, a history of trauma, or stress over an upcoming event can preclude the smooth flow of *qi* in the body and the ability to function in or outside of a therapy situation. Couples with a basically good relationship can find that relationship threatened when faced with financial worries or the birth of a child.
2. *It defends the body.* *Qi*, particularly antipathogenic *qi*, serves a protective function. It is responsible for keeping pathogens outside of the body and for fighting those that enter. Defensive *qi* thus serves the same function that the immune system does in Western medicine, but its conceptualization in Eastern physiology goes even further. The protective nature of *qi* acts like an organic sieve at the body's surface. It can screen incoming elements and decide whether or not they should be accepted. If the stimulus is unwanted, defensive *qi* closes off the entry and acts as a barrier. Since this system does not separate emotional and physical factors, this protective capacity also operates in interpersonal relationships. Individuals who barricade themselves against social or emotional involvement have overprotective *qi* functions. Those who fail to discriminate appropriate from inappropriate interpersonal interactions have a defensive system that is not sufficiently active. Enmeshment, disengagement, nymphomania, or agoraphobia could all be products of improperly functioning defensive *qi*.

Mary was a single mother with two children, nine-year-old Bernard and eight-year-old Joseph. Because she was adamant in her desire to keep unwanted influences away from her children, she refused to open the door to visitors or even to answer the telephone. When the school complained of the boys' truancy, the court ordered her to seek therapy, and she complied out of fear that the boys would be taken away from her if she didn't do so. Mary's twin sister, Gwen, wrote to the therapist, supporting her sister's right to raise her children as she saw fit. Gwen described their upbringing as severely traumatic, and said that she felt that if her sister wanted to protect her children in turn, she should be given the chance. The therapist used Mary's need for privacy and protection to drive the therapy. He suggested that her current actions made her life a fishbowl, with educational and social welfare agencies constantly peering in. She decided to allow the boys to attend school for a trial period, with the agreement that if she felt they were being traumatized in any way, she could apply for home schooling. In return, the court would suspend active monitoring of the family.

3. *It is the source of harmonious transformations*. *Qi* provides the mechanism to create change. Whether it's air from the outside being turned into usable energy within the body, food being changed into absorbable nutrients, or self-actualization, *qi* is the catalyst for the process. For any meaningful transformations to occur, sufficient levels of *qi* must be present.
4. *It serves a checking function*. For bodily activity to proceed smoothly, everything must be in its proper place. Blood must stay in its vessels, urine and sperm must be released only when desired, and tears and sweat must be held in check until needed. When *qi* is not functioning properly, organs prolapse, enuresis occurs, sperm ejaculates prematurely, and sweating takes place for no reason. The same applies to emotional symptoms. Anger that comes from nowhere, uncontrollable crying, or an inability to "keep it together" could all be symptomatic of *qi*'s not fulfilling its checking function.
5. *It warms the body and maintains heat*. If *qi* is circulating smoothly in the body, warmth is carried to all of the limbs and organs. Cold hands and feet indicate that *qi* flow into those areas is poor. A rigid, unresponsive demeanor or being overly sensitive to chilly weather is also a sign that not enough of the warming quality of *qi* is present.

### Xue

*Xue* ("shway") is most typically translated as "blood," but once again, this is an oversimplification. *Xue* is a more material element than *qi* and is primarily composed of fluids, the nourishing components obtained from food, and the *qi* obtained from breathing. This is very similar to the Western concept that blood is composed of fluids and nutrients oxygenated by the lungs. *Xue*, like blood, is propelled through the body by the heart, but unlike its Western counterpart, it moves not only inside the blood vessels, but also through the meridians, tissues, and organs. A sufficient level of *xue* is necessary for healthy functioning, but its quality is also important.

*Xue* serves three primary functions in the body.

1. *It nourishes the body*. *Xue* is responsible for carrying nutrients throughout the body. If the limbs or organs are undernourished, it is because of low levels or a poor quality of *xue*. Deficiencies of muscle tone or function, withered limbs, malnutrition, and poor coordination could all be considered manifestations of a problem with *xue*. Blurred vision signifies that *xue* is not sufficiently nourishing the eyes.
2. *It moistens the body*. Excessive dryness is also indicative of poor *xue* function. Dry eyes, skin, and hair can be produced by insufficient *xue* levels. Similarly, the decrease in vaginal lubrication seen during menopause is related to a reduction in the quality of *xue* at that time.
3. *It is integrally related to mental activities and health*. It is this function of *xue* that is most relevant to psychotherapy. In order for mental functioning to proceed smoothly, the mind must be nourished and moistened. If *xue* is insufficient or its quality is poor, such problems as insomnia and memory loss can result, simply because the mind is not receiving enough nourishment. Thought disorders are also felt to be a product of low levels of *xue* in the mind, and mania is produced because the moistening properties of *xue* are deficient. The disoriented mental processes of individuals after a stroke or head trauma are thought to be the result of the disrupted flow of *xue* to the brain. This conceptualization is not that different from that of Western medicine, which describes cerebral accidents as a loss of oxygen to the brain.

In Eastern healing systems, the excessive loss of *xue* owing to hemorrhage from bleeding ulcers or in childbirth leads to difficulties involving all three of its primary functions; it can also produce problems with *qi* levels, since *xue* carries nutritive energy in its fluids.

Barbara had been finding life difficult since the birth of her baby. She didn't feel as though she could move a muscle and every chore she performed took effort. Her hair fell lank and lifeless, her skin was sallow, and there were patches of dry, scaly areas on her legs.

What bothered Barbara most was that she couldn't remember simple things, such as whether she had fed the baby, cooked dinner, or had done the wash. She wasn't sleeping well at night, even though her husband, Greg, attended to the baby when she woke. Barbara found the baby's crying irritating, and as she often didn't have the energy to comfort the child, she usually would just go into the backyard to get away from the noise.

***Jing***

If *yuan qi* is the energy we inherit from our parents, *jing* is the more substantial essence we receive from them. *Jing* is comparable, in Western terms, to the genetic plan. It is the basis for our potential and growth. Like *yuan qi*, it must be protected and preserved, since our parents pass on only a basic amount to us. The quality of *jing* that a parent transmits declines with successive offspring. Firstborn children generally get the best-grade *jing*, with future siblings receiving an inferior product.

*Jing* is the basis for reproduction and development. The aging of an individual proceeds along the path set up by *jing*, from infancy, to childhood, adolescence, adulthood, and old age. Problems with insufficient development (mental retardation) or premature aging (early senility or graying of the hair) are felt to be related to poor-quality *jing*. While people cannot alter the nature of the *jing* given to them by their parents, they can maximize acquisition of postnatal *jing*.

Acquired *jing* is cultivated through healthy living—eating right, sleeping well, and enjoying a sensible lifestyle. Among the most significant ways to lose *jing* are through orgasm in men and childbirth in women. Although women don't release *jing* with orgasm, men lose *jing* each time they ejaculate. Some Taoist sex guides suggest that women actually accumulate the *jing* that men release during sex. Men, therefore, need to cultivate an extremely healthy lifestyle if they want to have frequent ejaculations.

At a conference on Eastern healing, a 95-year-old practitioner from China spoke on longevity, emphasizing moderation in all things. Although a nonagenarian, the man bounded onto the stage, looking not a day over 50. During the talk, a young man asked him whether the methods he was promoting also allowed him to have sex frequently, or whether he worried about loss of *jing*. His answer, as translated: "My methods work well. I doubt you could keep up!"

If *jing* is at an adequate level, the body functions well, the organs are healthy, aging effects are minimal, and there is growth on all levels. If too much *jing* is being consumed, organs and bones fall apart, there are signs of premature aging, and the level of personal potential is diminished.

Jack, a 34-year-old stockbroker, presented for treatment because he had begun to have panic attacks. Jack was highly successful in his work, and relentlessly pursued his goal of achieving a wealthy retirement by the age of 40. He didn't want any permanent relationships in his life that might slow him down, but Jack loved to party, and he frequently maintained intimate involvements with up to four women at a time. A typical day for him would be to wake at 4 A.M. to catch early stock reports from around the world, leave for the office by 6, work 12 hours, and then head for a bar after work, and someone's bed later on. Jack's pace was recently being hampered by sudden rushes of panic, accompanied by palpitations, sweating, and difficulty in breathing. The bouts would only last about two minutes, but he was becoming apprehensive, dreading their arrival. Jack was also annoyed because he didn't have his usual energy. His back ached when he was at his desk, and his hearing was less acute than normal.

### *Shen*

*Shen* is spirit, will, and sense. It is composed of *jing*, but it is actually the form through which that essence is expressed. *Shen* is reflected in one's outward appearance—the gloss of the skin and the sparkle in the eye. It is essentially the organizing and transformative influence that determines and upholds an individual's character. It is an expression of who you are, how you are, and where you are going.

If *qi* is the source of movement, then *shen* is the vitality, force, and direction behind the movement. It is a reflection of the interior psyche. When discussing something stimulating, a person shines with animation.

If one has lost hope and confidence, one's *shen* is subdued and dull. In Eastern medicine, a practitioner is able to determine how easily a person can be treated by assessing how intact his or her *shen* is. People with complex symptoms and extensive histories of problems still have a good prognosis if their eyes sparkle. Patients with minor problems but a depressed *shen* are much harder to treat.

In Eastern healing, there is also a condition known as "false" *shen*. This is commonly seen in terminally ill patients prior to death. A person who had been listless and noncommunicative will sometimes perk up and chat animatedly with loved ones just before dying. It is felt to be a final rallying of the spirit, a chance to say goodbye and to grasp life before it disappears.

In therapy, a less final, but still serious, form of false *shen* is seen in individuals who project an aura of confidence, sparkle, assurance, or charm that is not an accurate reflection of what is happening within. The charismatic, outward glow masks an interior marked by doubt, turmoil, or insecurity. One such client presented for therapy because she was exhausted from trying to control a stutter. She was terrified that someone would find out that she had a speech dysfluency, and so she kept it under rigid control, whether at work or with her family or friends. The price of maintaining such vigilance was beginning to take its toll, and she would find herself weeping for no reason whenever she was alone.

Psychopathic personalities can also be seen as deliberately manipulating their *shen*. Their outward façade can be charming, concealing a far darker side. At other times, a powerful *shen* can be used to manipulate others in an interpersonal situation. Consider the case of Jerry and Helen, and the opposite ways in which *shen* became manifest in their relationship.

Jerry, 42 years old, used his charisma to become a successful entrepreneur. People were engaged by his level of energy and charm to the point that they would rush into business arrangements with him. He always accomplished what he set out to accomplish and was held in high esteem by customers and colleagues.

Jerry attended therapy with his ex-wife, Helen, and their two children. Helen said that Jerry was so persuasive in his arguments that she had begun to doubt her ability as a mother. He had convinced Helen that it was all right for him to beat their children, until her mother stepped in and stopped it. Helen was dispirited, saying that she felt incapable of taking any action, because she didn't trust her own judgment. She often yielded to Jerry because he seemed so certain and secure.

## In Conclusion

The building blocks of Eastern healing—*qi*, *xue*, *jing*, and *shen*—have implications for psychotherapy. In subsequent chapters, these concepts will be discussed in terms of diagnosis and treatment.

# CHAPTER TWO

## Differential Diagnosis

■

*Once the whole is divided, the parts need*
*names.*
*There are already enough names.*
*One must know when to stop.*

—*Lao-tzu*

Fundamental to Eastern healing is the development of a differential diagnosis, the process by which a practitioner collates information from a variety of sources to formulate a statement that defines a patient at that point in time. As in psychotherapy, diagnosis in Eastern medicine is both an art and a science. In both systems, the practitioner must examine the patient and compare his or her pattern against an established template. Whereas a therapist might label a client as bipolar, disengaged, or suffering from a posttraumatic stress syndrome, an acupuncturist might see the person as having phlegm misting the heart, dampness in the spleen, or deranged *qi*. The differences between the diagnostic terms, however, extend beyond the terminologies used by the two systems.

Eastern medicine uses a diagnosis as a prescription for treatment. By naming the condition, a hypothesis is established that allows the practitioner to follow a course of action. The diagnosis is never considered solid or immutable. A patient might have liver fire rising, but he or she never *is* liver fire rising. This differs radically from diagnoses that are generated by the fourth edition of the *Diagnostic and Statistical Manual of Mental Disorders* (DSM-IV), where the client is schizophrenic, has attention-deficit/hyperactivity disorder (ADHD), or is obsessive-compulsive. In Eastern healing, the condition is felt to be an interplay among current or past environmental events, the antipathogenic *qi* of the individual, and the person's constitutional strengths and weaknesses. It is not a definition of who that patient is or is likely to become.

If a differential diagnosis is perceived as a working hypothesis, the practitioner is able to try a likely course of treatment, evaluate its impact on the client, and then adjust either the treatment plan or the diagnosis. Change can come slowly or rapidly, but both the diagnosis and the course of treatment are continually assessed for their validity and usefulness. There are times when a patient's diagnostic category actually changes during a single session due to the effect of the treatment.

Psychotherapeutic diagnoses are not that flexible. A schizophrenic client who spontaneously stops having hallucinations, delusions, or thought disorder commonly is seen as being "in remission." It as if the disorder is lurking there, inextricably intertwined with the person's genetic code, waiting to make another appearance. If the client stays normal for an extended time, the original diagnosis is questioned as to its accuracy.

Diagnoses that are fixed and reified immobilize both patients and therapists. Clients become unable to conceptualize themselves as independent of the disorder even if an aspect of their functioning has no relation to that problem. A newspaper article on adult ADD (*Sunday Star-Times*, March 12, 1995) described a man who was unable to stay faithful to his wife and attributed this to his inability to concentrate on one thing for very long. The man presented himself as a helpless victim of the exigencies of his disorder. Although this particular reframing may have been an attempt to escape the wrath of a spouse, it is common in clients who find themselves labeled with a psychiatric diagnosis. Responsibility, effort, and the capacity to change are hobbled by their syndrome.

Therapists are equally nearsighted when a client's diagnosis becomes reality. All expectations of successful resolution disappear, and maintenance and containment become the therapeutic goals. The therapist works to maximize functioning within the context of the syndrome rather than anticipating its transformation. Someone with major depression can do well or poorly, but the shadow is always there.

Many psychotherapists have rebelled against the medical model of diagnosis. They refuse to label clients, taking each session as an independent event, and trying to resolve their clients' issues in an active, nonjudgmental way. By refusing to diagnose on any level, however, therapists allow the therapy to be driven by the client, or the moment, without a defined goal.

Some therapists operate in a manner similar to that of the Eastern system. Based on information provided by the client and his or her behavior during sessions, the therapist develops a working hypothesis of what the presenting and underlying issues are and how they can best be addressed. Therapy proceeds toward this goal while continually reassessing the accuracy of the hypothesis and the effectiveness of the plan. Diagnosis emerges as a constructive tool, rather than as an end point or limitation.

## Eastern Diagnostics

Eastern healing uses four primary avenues of gathering information:

1. Looking
2. Listening and smelling (the same word in Chinese)
3. Asking
4. Touching

### *Looking*

Both Eastern medical practitioners and psychotherapists gain an initial impression of clients from their appearance. The client's *shen* is readily observed at the first meeting. Clients also convey information by their body language, and whether a client sits up straight, is curled forward, runs around the room, or slumps in a chair provides useful data for both types of practitioner.

In Eastern medicine, there are also several other ways of learning about clients by looking. Changes in the client's skin tone, for example, can be related to organ dysfunction. Eastern medical practitioners also use tongue diagnosis to assess the state of the client. By looking at the shape and color of the tongue, the type of coating, and how much moisture is present, a practitioner can gather information about the physiological workings of the body.

### *Listening and Smelling*

Both Eastern healers and psychotherapists learn about their clients by listening to how they communicate. A person who speaks in a low, quiet voice is likely to have problems that are very different from those presented by someone who continually shouts or is boisterous. Clients using incoherent speech or random utterances would be of concern to either practitioner. Eastern healers also listen to the pattern of breathing as a way to identify *qi* difficulties or the presence of phlegm, and they are inquisitive about odors emanating from the patient, including the smell of feces and urine, as this information helps in formulating a diagnosis.

### *Asking*

Obviously, the category that psychotherapy and Eastern medicine have most in common is "asking." Both inquire about relevant information from the client's past, as well as from present circumstances. In addition, a practitioner of Eastern medicine might question a client about chills and fever, patterns of perspiration, appetite and thirst, defecation and urination, sleeping patterns, or menses and sexual function. Like the psychotherapist, the practitioner would also make specific inquiries into the presenting problem, what makes it better or worse, and how often it occurs.

### *Touching*

An Eastern medical practitioner certainly has more latitude to gain information about clients by touching than does a psychotherapist. The most important aspect of palpation is taking the pulse. While there are numerous systems of pulse diagnosis in Eastern medicine, all depend on taking pulses at the radial artery on the wrist. Usually three fingers are laid on the client's arm, with the practitioner's pressing both lightly and more heavily. By assessing the pulses on each arm, the healer can determine the state of *qi* and *xue* in the body, the presence of pathogens, and the health of the organs. Other aspects of palpation include touching key points on the body to determine whether or not they are sensitive and examining the abdomen by pressing.

■

Although the diagnostic methods used in Eastern healing often differ from those of psychotherapy, they serve the same goal. Both practitioners seek to understand the client's pattern of difficulty in order to facilitate resolution of the problem. The following three cases, in which the patients were seen by both a psychotherapist and an Eastern medical practitioner, are presented so that the two approaches to diagnosis can be compared.

### *Evelyn*

Evelyn was referred for treatment by her physician because of serious pain secondary to her bone cancer. When Evelyn showed up for her appointment, it was obvious that she was experiencing a high level of discomfort that affected her ability to move. Her emotional outlook was extremely bright, however. Evelyn said that the doctors predicted that she would be dead by April, but she was determined to see the birth of her first grandchild in October. She was also driven to stay active in her work and social life. Evelyn had refused high doses of pain medication because she felt they impaired her ability to achieve her other goals.

The therapist chatted with Evelyn about her expectations of life and of therapy. They decided that she would profit most from hypnosis to help her with managing her pain. She entered trance easily and suggestions were offered to enable her to control her pain more successfully. Eventually, the hypnosis shifted to developing images of health and well-being.

Evelyn presented a similar demeanor when visiting the Eastern medical practitioner. Her bright *shen* indicated a considerable reserve of source *qi*, despite the effects of the cancer on her body. Black circles under her eyes and the pallor of her skin pointed to problems with her kidney energetics. Evelyn's pulse confirmed this and indicated high levels of water stagnation and pain. Palpation of her abdomen revealed the presence of nodules and edema. Examination of her tongue showed signs of fluid involvement and depleted *qi*, but also a solid core of resources. She was diagnosed as having insufficient Kidney and Spleen *qi*, leading to an accumulation of phlegm damp in the interior. She was given acupuncture and an appropriate herbal remedy.

Because of the seriousness of her problems, Evelyn was seen on a twice-weekly basis by both therapists for a month. She reported a significant decrease in pain after the first sessions, and by the end of the month, she felt able to manage the pain through self-hypnosis. She continued with the herbal treatments for the following two years, seeing not only the birth of her grandchild, but also his first birthday.

### *Tommy*

Tommy, the 16-year-old who had begun to have blackouts while he was running, was discussed briefly in the Introduction. As a result of his blackouts, his general practitioner referred him for neurological examination but neither his electroencephalogram nor his CAT scan revealed significant findings. When Tommy's blackouts began to increase, his physician referred him to the inpatient child and adolescent unit at the hospital for closer examination. In speaking with a psychiatrist, Tommy mentioned that during one of his blackouts, he heard a voice, which he called "Phil," speak to him. The voice did not request or discuss anything specific. Because of the lack of hard neurological evidence to support a medical diagnosis, the team of psychiatrists determined that Tommy had a dissociative disorder and referred him to the appropriate outpatient mental health facility.

Tommy was next interviewed by a psychiatrist at the outpatient clinic. The psychiatrist concluded that Tommy was developing his symptoms in response to family turmoil, and so referred him to a family therapist. When the therapist met with Tommy and his parents, the parents reported that prior to the past few months, there had been some tension in their marriage. Whenever his parents argued, Tommy frequently would side with his mother. Tommy admitted that he felt uncomfortable when his parents fought, but that he did not feel that this was producing his blackouts. His mother added that their marriage problems had been resolved over the past three months, but that Tommy's problems were getting worse. The father was concerned about Tommy's diagnosis by the psychiatrists, as he felt that the cause of the blackouts was medical—although, except for the general practitioner, none of the medical personnel were willing to consider this possibility.

The therapist worked with the family over the next three weeks, addressing the alienation of Tommy and his father and coordinating the parents with regard to Tommy's behavior. They felt that they all were interacting much more positively with each other, but Tommy continued to have blackouts.

The family decided to try acupuncture treatment for Tommy. The acpuncturist saw Tommy as a frail-looking, but athletic youth, with pallid skin and dark circles under his eyes. His pulse was thready and fast, and his tongue indicated a deficiency of both *qi* and *xue*. Tommy reported difficulty in sleeping and occasional dizzy spells. He also indicated a history of dull headaches and a lack of energy in the afternoon. Further inquiry revealed that Tommy's blackouts usually occurred after he had participated in a series of excessively strenuous activities (for example, a 15-mile run followed the next day by a rock-climbing excursion, with an all-night party in between). They also seemed to be exacerbated when he ate junk food.

Tommy was diagnosed as having deficient *qi* and *xue*. Acupuncture focused on restoring good energy circulation, but it was secondary to recommendations that Tommy change his lifestyle and diet. While Tommy acknowledged that he felt better as a result of the acupuncture, he was unwilling to modify his schedule or nutritional intake. Because his system was inherently depleted, there was no way for acupuncture alone to restore Tommy's energy. A referral back to the family therapist was suggested to help with compliance.

Tommy's family chose to return to their general practitioner instead, who again referred Tommy to the outpatient psychiatrist. He now diagnosed Tommy as having a conversion reaction, since no signs of dissociative behavior were present. The psychiatrist did not feel that there was any appropriate medication, so he suggested that Tommy's condition be "watched" for further developments.

#### *Karen*

Karen, 14 years old, presented with a history of headaches so severe that she had not been able to attend school for six months. She was accompanied to her acupuncture treatment by her mother, although Karen insisted that the mother remain in the waiting room. Karen was extremely mature for her age, dressing and acting like a prim adult woman. In a formal manner, she detailed the history of her illness. Her headaches had begun when she was a young child. Numerous treatments had been attempted, including a visit to a leading national pain clinic. Pharmacological intervention, biofeedback, and stress-reduction plans had proved equally unsuccessful. Karen did not feel comfortable in school, so she had stopped attending, pursuing her education through independent study.

Differential diagnosis revealed some stagnation of *qi* and a deficiency of *xue*, but no major signs of pathology. Karen did not show any sensitivity upon palpation, and the only other significant problems in her history seemed related to her sleep patterns. Appetite and color were good, with no difficulties with elimination or her menses. Before acupuncture treatment was initiated, Karen was asked to rate her pain on a scale of 1 to 10. The practitioner was surprised when Karen rated it as only a 5. When asked whether this was a typical level for her, she stated that the pain rarely got worse than that and was often less. Karen did not feel that it was odd that mild to moderate pain was having such a significant impact on her life.

Acupuncture treatment centered on restoring the smooth flow of *qi*, reducing Karen's pain and improving her sleep. She reported a reduction of pain to a 2 during treatment. At the next appointment, Karen said that she had slept better during the interval between sessions. After several treatments, when she began to despair because her pain was not completely gone, even though it had been reduced to a mild level, she was referred to a psychotherapist for assistance.

Once again, Karen was accompanied to the session by her mother, but she refused to allow her to come into the room even to meet the therapist. Karen detailed the history of her headaches willingly. She was very evasive about her home situation, although she alluded to her mother as being incompetent and to her father as a knight in shining armor. She would not consider bringing her family into therapy and insisted that all she wanted was help with her pain. The therapist used hypnosis with Karen, although it was difficult to produce much change since she had rated her pain as a 3 at the beginning of the session. At their next meeting, the therapist attempted to discuss matters other than headaches with Karen, but she refused. The therapist asked her if he could call her parents to talk about a treatment plan, and she agreed. When the therapist telephoned Karen's father that evening, he was told that Karen did not wish to continue therapy on any level. When the therapist suggested that she might be able to return to school if the family worked together toward that goal, the father terminated the conversation.

## In Conclusion

While there are fundamental differences between the ways in which psychotherapists and Eastern healers collect information, they are both best served by developing a differential diagnosis. This working hypothesis can assist in formulating a plan for treatment and provide guidelines for assessing success without permanently locking the client into a particular syndrome.

## Part Two

# THE EIGHT PRINCIPLES

*Therefore having and not having arise together.*
*Difficult and easy complement each other.*
*Long and short contrast each other.*
*High and low rest upon each other.*
*Voice and sound harmonize each other.*
*Front and back follow one another.*

*—Lao-tzu*

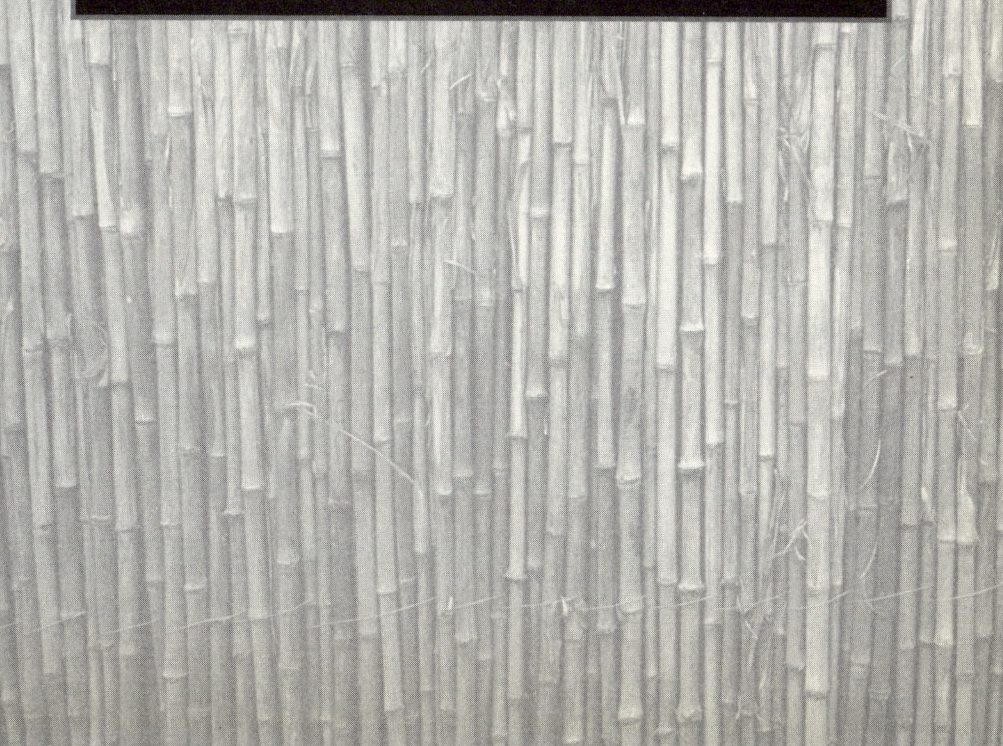

At the heart of Eastern healing is a dichotomous system known as the eight principles. By determining where a patient falls in relation to the four diagnostic pairs (*yin/yang*, hot/cold, internal/external, deficiency/excess), a proper treatment can be formulated.

*Yin* and *yang* are the overriding duality. In traditional writing, *yin* is compared to the shady side of a hill and *yang* to the sunny slope. The hill is a single unit of nature, indivisible without creating havoc. The cool, darker aspects of the shady side contrast markedly with the warmth and light on the other slope, but they are fundamentally part of the same hill. The qualities of the two sides of the hill are transformatory, not static. As the sun moves across the sky, the sunny side becomes dark, the shady side becomes bright. In the same way, the eight principles are not fixed attributes, but relational ones.

# CHAPTER THREE

## *Yin* and *Yang*

■

*Under heaven all can see beauty as beau-*
*ty only because there is ugliness.*
*All can know good as good only because*
*there is evil.*

*—Lao-tzu*

The meaning of *yin* and *yang* can best be understood within the symbol of the *taiqitu* ("tye-chee-too"), the image of great polarity. This symbol, adopted by atomic regulatory agencies and surfware manufacturers, stands as a metaphor for the dynamics of the dichotomy. It was originally colored red and blue, since the aspects of *yang* were compared to fire and of *yin* to water, and turned on its side. Over the years, perhaps because life became more black and white, the symbol shifted into the colors and position shown in Figure 3.1.

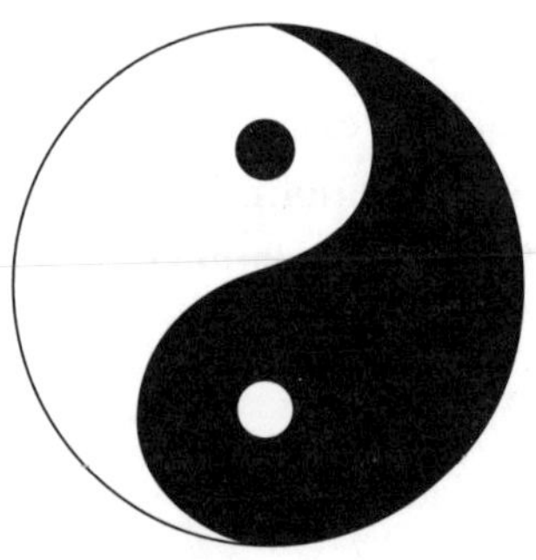

**Figure 3.1.** *Taiqitu.*

The meaning of the *taiqitu* is linked to four primary relationships between *yin* and *yang*.

### *Opposition of Yin and Yang*

All of nature can be divided into *yin* and *yang* components. *Yin*, the black side of the symbol, possesses the qualities of water (substance, fluidity, downward flow, coolness, dampness), and *yang*, the white side of the symbol, has the attributes of fire (warmth, movement, upward motion, insubstantiality). Table 3.1 lists some qualities of *yin* and *yang* used by Eastern medicine.

| ***YIN*** | ***YANG*** |
|---|---|
| Water | Fire |
| Cold | Hot |
| Night | Day |
| Fall/winter | Spring/summer |
| Female | Male |
| Heavier | Lighter |
| Dull | Bright |
| Damp | Dry |
| Falling | Rising |
| Static | Moving |
| Left | Right |
| Dull pain | Sharp pain |
| Chronic | Acute |
| Interior | Exterior |
| Front of the body | Back of the body |
| Trunk | Limbs |
| *Xue* | *Qi* |
| Organs | Meridians |
| Flaccidity | Spasm |
| Empty | Full |
| Bones | Skin |
| Deficiency | Excess |
| Lower | Higher |

**Table 3.1.** *Examples of* Yin *and* Yang *Characteristics in Eastern Healing*

Larger, louder, and more outgoing people with severe headaches or skin disruptions would be *yang*. Problems involving fluids in the body, difficulties that occur at night, and organ prolapse would all be *yin*. Table 3.2 presents similar pairs of terms from psychotherapy.

| ***YIN*** | ***YANG*** |
|---|---|
| Dependent | Independent |
| Criticism | Praise |
| Depression | Mania |
| Frigid | Hypersexual |
| Withdrawn | Gregarious |
| Enmeshed | Disengaged |
| Restrained | Exuberant |
| Static | Changing |
| Passive | Aggressive |
| Regression | Development |
| Denial | Overindulgence |
| Compliant | Defiant |
| Phobic | Fearless |
| Reflective | Directive |
| Calm | Anxious |
| Relapse | Progress |
| Relaxation | Stress |
| Immobility | Hyperactivity |
| Anorexia | Overeating |
| Unconscious | Conscious |
| Certain | Ambivalent |
| Intrapersonal | Interpersonal |
| Focused | Distractible |
| Rule-bound | Free-wheeling |
| Methodical | Spontaneous |

**Table 3.2.** *Examples of* Yin *and* Yang *Characteristics in Psychotherapy*

Clients who are more violent, active, or independent would have a preponderance of *yang*. Those who have chronic problems, depressed affect, or are more reflective would be *yin*.

Balance and health result when both elements are present in opposition. An individual needs to be able to move, but also benefits from quiet.

Disharmony results when one of the factors, *yin* or *yang*, is present in a disproportionate amount. In Eastern healing, diagnosis and treatment depend on determining the relevant preponderance of the two factors. Neither quality is considered positive or negative, better or worse; the existence of both is necessary to healthy functioning.

In psychotherapy, we tend to be more judgmental. Such qualities as adaptability, growth, and nurturance are generally seen as positive, whereas hostility, stagnation, and inflexibility are perceived negatively. The reality, however, is that any of these features could be either helpful or counterproductive in a given context. Someone who adapts to any situation may have difficulty feeling grounded, and a parent who won't allow a 25-year-old son to leave home might be using nurturance in an unhelpful way. It could be perfectly appropriate to be hostile to an attacker, and stagnation could be framed as the capacity to stay still long enough to explore issues thoroughly.

The meaning of any characteristic is found within its context; there is no inherent value. In fact, whether something is *yin* or *yang* is relative and changing. For example, if greater size is a *yang* construct, you might be *yang* in relation to an infant but *yin* in relation to a player from the NBA. Water is generally perceived as a *yin* element, but pounding ocean waves have many *yang* features. The message of the *taiqitu* is that it is important to think relationally rather than statically.

Problems usually arise when one aspect dominates the other. A bipolar condition could be seen as an alternation between too much *yang* (mania, rushing around, overactivity) and too much *yin* (depression, lack of movement, depressed affect). In individuals with more balance, excessive movement is checked by a cooling *yin* quality and inaction is prodded by activity.

The *taiqitu* demonstrates the importance of balance between the factors in two ways. First, to create and make the circle complete, compensatory levels of *yin* and *yang* must be present. Second, in each half of the symbol, there is another circle of the opposite factor, a dot of white in the black and of black in the white. In the depths of *yin*, you find a base of *yang*; in the core of *yang*, there is an element of *yin*. Although one or the other can predominate at a given time, both are always present.

### *Interdependence of Yin and Yang*

Although *yin* and *yang* are opposites, they are also complementary. The existence of one depends on the presence of the other. Philosophy has struggled with this issue of duality for thousands of years, arguing whether the existence of goodness depends on evil, joy on sadness, or health on illness. Leaving the debate aside, in functional systems, it seems that *yin* and *yang* features are usually interdependent. In Eastern medicine, *xue*, a *yin* factor, cannot move without *qi*, a *yang* factor. Similarly, the production of *qi* (*yang*) depends on the healthy functioning of the organs (*yin*) that make it.

In many relationships, one person's characteristics drive the behavior of the other. This can be a good fit or a pathological interaction. In a therapy situation, for instance, a client who prefers to give a therapist total control matches well with a therapist who likes to be directive. The opposition of their stances creates a good working relationship. In some interactions, however, participants get locked into an interdependence that is less healthy.

Ann and Dave, married for 18 years, presented for therapy. Ann complained that she was tired of providing all of the emotional support in the relationship. She said that Dave was self-indulgent and relied on everyone else, especially Ann, to solve his problems. The couple described a cycle in which the more passive Dave became, the more active a role Ann assumed. If things didn't work out the way he wanted, Dave struck out at everyone, especially his wife. Ann generally took the blame, and then increased her attempts to help.

Ann stated that the couple's interactions had become so difficult and burdensome that she felt they needed to separate. Even then, Ann wanted to help Dave find a suitable apartment and to furnish it for him. She offered to clean it once a week and to do his grocery shopping. When Dave became angry about the separation and cruel about Ann's pandering to him, Ann offered to stay with him and apologized for her actions.

In the course of therapy, Ann and Dave worked to achieve a more balanced independence. After jointly agreeing to a separation, Ann began to pursue interests she had abandoned during her marriage and developed a career. Dave eventually was able to make his own choices and to respond to his family in a nonaccusatory manner.

***Intertransforming Relationship of Yin and Yang***

In nature, there is a natural progression of *yin* to *yang* and *yang* to *yin*. Night becomes day and day drifts into night. The seasons of the year follow a similar progression, with the cold of winter yielding to the warmth of spring, the heat of summer shifting to the cool of autumn. Similar patterns can be seen in people. Bouts of excessive motion are followed by the quiet of exhaustion. Work seems more enticing after a restful holiday.

In the *taiqitu*, the transformation of one aspect to another takes place when either *yang* or *yin* has reached its peak. If one follows the course of *yin*, for example, from a small tail of black to a full lobe, one can see that the transformation to *yang* happens when *yin* is at its highest levels. The warmth of spring comes after the cold of winter, not the coolness of autumn. For one aspect to transform into the other, an extreme level needs to be reached. Consider febrile diseases. When the fever reaches its zenith, the situation changes radically, and the patient often lies freezing beneath the covers.

This transformation is also seen in the therapeutic milieu. Many clients present for therapy only after their situation has reached a sufficiently intolerable level. Clients in crisis are sometimes the easiest to help because the extremity of their problem makes them more amenable to suggestions. Individuals who are stuck in the bog of inertia or ambivalence need much more energy to move toward resolution.

The intertransforming of *yin* and *yang* can also be seen in therapy situations where a client's radical behavior switches to a similarly extreme opposite pattern.

> Sixteen-year-old Bill was always getting into trouble. His school complained about his behavior and lack of academic effort. He was disruptive at home and frequently fought with his mother, sometimes even threatening her with violence. His father had been sent to prison for manslaughter when Bill was a baby. The school referred the family for therapy after Bill was expelled for setting books on fire in the library.
>
> During the first month of therapy, Bill's behavior changed radically. He became very polite to his mother and began attending bible study classes at his church. A month later, Bill was spending his free time on street corners downtown, preaching the gospel with parishioners from his church. The

only time he was disruptive at home was when he became frustrated because his mother did not attend church more regularly. By the end of therapy, Bill had enrolled in a preministry program and was running groups for teenagers, at which he talked about the dangers of alcohol and drugs and the need for a good education.

The transformation of *yin* to *yang* can also happen interpersonally. Dyadic relationships frequently cycle from one extreme to the other. Violent relationships often build up to an eruption, and then, once the confrontation has taken place, conciliation and calm follow. The transformation of *yin* to *yang* can also occur across generations.

Tim, a 31-year-old youth worker, presented for therapy because he was conflicted in his relationships with his family. Having grown up with an alcoholic father and a passive mother, he described his family life as a series of incidents, in which his father would come home drunk in an abusive and contentious mood, Tim would hide in his room, and his mother would make excuses for his father or deny that there was a problem. Tim's older brother, Frank, would defend the father, praising his hard work, and generally feeling sorry for him.

Tim said that now, as an adult, he was unable to be around anyone who was drinking, as it made him nauseous to watch them. He realized that this limited his social life, since attending weddings, office parties, or even a ball game would precipitate his feeling ill. Tim doesn't speak to his father, although he visits his mother, whose Alzheimer's disease has confined her to a nursing home. He continually preaches to Frank, who is unemployed and drinks heavily, about the dangers of winding up like their father.

### *Interconsuming/Intersupporting Relationship of Yin and Yang*

In this sense, consuming refers to a loss or weakening and supporting to gaining or strengthening. If you look at the line that runs down the middle of the *taiqitu*, you see that the relationship of *yin* and *yang* is not fixed, but fluctuates. Whenever there is more of one, there is less of the other. The metaphor of the symbol is very different from one where a circle would be bisected evenly into two halves. Within the *taiqitu*, there is movement in the relationship of *yin* and *yang*, and the predominance of one ensures the decrease of the other.

This pattern of gain and loss is normal as long as it does not become too extreme. For example, if you become warm from indulging in exercise, you can easily compensate for the increase of *yang* by drinking *yin* fluids. If the body gets overly hot from a fever, however, the extreme heat consumes fluids drastically, and it is more difficult to replace the loss of *yin*. Eating cold or raw food (ice cream, salad, fruit) requires the body to use heat to digest it. During the summer, the loss of *yang* from processing the food is not a problem. In the winter, however, there might be an insufficient level of heat present and eating cold foods results in poor digestion.

The ebb and flow of *yin* and *yang* can often be seen during the course of therapy. At times, clients will take a more active role; at other points, they may be withdrawn and passive. The therapeutic exchange works best when the therapist can adapt to the changing stances of the client, adjusting his or her position to compensate for the fluctuation.

> June, 31 years old, came to therapy agitated and angry. Her boyfriend of two years had left her for another woman. June was very upset and complained about the injustice of what had happened. Whenever the therapist tried to interject to gain clarification or gather information, June became irate, berating the therapist for being insensitive to the enormity of her problem. The therapist listened politely to June for half an hour. When she finally ran out of steam, he once again asked some questions and offered suggestions. June accepted the advice and asked for clarification of some of the proposed interventions. As she was setting up the next appointment, June apologized for her abrupt behavior earlier in the session.

The therapist needed to take a more receptive, *yin* stance during June's *yang* outburst at the beginning of the session. As her behavior transformed, the therapist was able to assume a more active position, eventually leading to balance by the end of the session.

# CHAPTER FOUR

## Internal and External

■

*Without going outside, you may know the whole world.*
*Without looking through the window, you may see the ways of heaven.*
*The farther you go, the less you know.*

*—Lao-tzu*

Whereas *yin* and *yang* describe the overall quality of a condition, the other six principles further refine the nature of the problem. The qualities of internal/external define the depth of the difficulty, whether it originates inside or outside of the body, and how it affects core functioning. By observing the direction of development in relation to the principles of internal/external, one can make decisions about prognosis and treatment.

### Etiology

In Eastern healing, external diseases are felt to be caused by the invasion of pathogens into the exterior of the body. There are six pernicious influences (wind, cold, heat, damp, dryness, and summer heat), environmental events so extreme or sudden that the body's antipathogenic *qi* is unable to defend against them. Being caught in a downpour or draft without proper clothing or protection puts an individual at risk for developing problems. Wind is the principal pathogen, driving other factors, such as cold and heat, into the body through entry points at the back of the neck (it is rare to see an acupuncturist out in inclement weather without a scarf).

As discussed in the Introduction, an individual whose antipathogenic *qi* is sufficiently strong can resist mild to moderate invasions of external influences. This idea is not that different from Western medicine's concept of bacteria and viruses, carried in air or water, that penetrate the body via the mouth, nose, and skin before encountering the immune system's army of white blood cells. If a person's resistance is strong, he or she remains healthy. A person whose immunological defenses are poor "catches" the disease.

Eastern healing perceives external problems, which are caused by factors outside the body and penetrate only the surface of the individual, as tending to be acute, even when extreme. Serious and chronic problems only develop when the antipathogenic *qi* fails to repel the pathogen and it penetrates to the interior of the body.

The same idea would also apply in psychotherapy, in that external events are only significant if they reach the interior of an individual or system. A divorce, loss of a job, and the death of a parent are potent external events that can create an acute disruption of functioning. Responses can be strong and emotional, but if the individual's antipathogenic *qi* is sufficiently robust, the effects are acute and not chronic. However, if the incident is able to penetrate to the internal core because one's defenses or coping strategies are inadequate, the consequences can be devastating and long term. Some individuals grieve for a while; others do so for a lifetime. The difference is the depth to which the death penetrates.

The difficulty with some psychodynamic systems is that they intensify an external experience to the point where it achieves sufficient power to transform into an internal phenomenon. For instance, if a therapist encourages a client to process a trauma by reliving it, the event can become so potent that the person's antipathogenic *qi* is unable to defend against the trauma and prevent it from being transferred to the interior. While the therapist's intent is to help the client by reducing repression and enabling the client to deal with the situation, the reality is that the intervention often magnifies and solidifies the trauma to the point that it penetrates deeper into the individual. In the Eastern system, a healer would attempt to strengthen one's antipathogenic *qi* while expelling the external event.

Although the progression of external factors to the interior is one cause of internal disease according to the Eastern system, there are other factors that directly influence internal processes. As mentioned in the Introduction, drastic emotional stress or change can disrupt internal function. Diet and exercise also have a significant impact on the internal health of the body. Eating is an important way to "keep the *qi* within pure and clean." Malnutrition or an inadequate intake of food limits the amount of *qi* that can be produced, and imbalanced diets affect the quality of both *qi* and *xue*. For the organs to function properly, sufficient amounts of nutritious substances must be ingested.

Poor intent during the preparation of food can actually decrease its value. A good cook is one who concentrates on each meal, endowing each morsel with *qi*. Thus, food is best when eaten at home or in a small restaurant where the cook can focus his or her energy on its preparation. Food that is frozen or microwaved is considered "wrecked" because its *qi* has been destroyed. One should also eat food with intent, concentrating on assimilating its energy into the body. For food to have its most positive impact, it should be grown with care, selected with care, prepared with attention, served fresh, and ingested with awareness.

Exercise and work are felt to have a major influence on the internal health of the body as well. If the body does not receive enough exercise, *qi* and *xue* begin to stagnate. A sufficient level of movement is needed to "stir the soup" so that everything moves harmoniously and nothing settles prematurely. If there is a lack of exercise and movement, stagnation of *qi* can take place, resulting in such problems as lassitude, depression, rumination, and irritability.

> Jerry, a therapist, realized that he felt better and less depressed about work whenever he regularly followed a running program. He was frustrated, however, by his inability to convince his depressed clients to try running also. His suggestions that they start exercising were usually ignored, because they were often so depressed that they didn't have the energy to get started. Jerry decided to overcome his clients' inertia by donning his running shoes and jogging with them, alternating therapy sessions with running, or combining the two. He got total compliance in this way, and his clients soon reported

an increase in energy and a decrease in their feelings of depression. Jerry also noticed that his clients were better able to address their issues and to follow other suggestions because they had the energy to do so. As a result, therapy proceeded more rapidly with these clients and with better results than with his depressed clients who were not running. As he eventually accumulated a number of clients who enjoyed running, Jerry formed a runners' group, initiating perhaps the first actively mobile depressed self-help group.

Too much exercise and work, however, consume *jing* and *qi*, resulting in a wasting of the body and declining organ function. Long-distance runners who follow schedules that are too rigorous to allow their bodies to recover sufficiently often experience serious difficulties with their bowels and hearts during their training and later in life. Workaholics often feel run down and are more susceptible to such problems as hypertension, insomnia, and gastric disturbances. For *qi* to flow smoothly, *jing* to be conserved, and *xue* to nourish the body, one must exercise in moderation—not too little, and not too much.

## Treatment

Since internal problems are more serious and chronic than are external difficulties, their treatment is usually more difficult and their prognosis poorer. Treating bulimia is harder than curing the indigestion caused by a holiday meal. Because of the relative severity and intractability of internal problems, Eastern healing protocols avoid pulling acute, external problems to a deeper level. In the same way, a psychotherapist is unlikely to suggest to a client that the reason he or she was snubbed by a coworker was that the client is unworthy of love, but is much more likely to help the client frame it as a contextual event.

If a problem penetrates to an internal level, several strategies for treatment are available. First, the severity of the difficulty and its degree of impact need to be assessed. A problem that causes minimal disruption can often be handled by strengthening other compensatory systems in the body. At other times, treatment might require bringing the problem back to the exterior where it can be handled more effectively.

Sam came to therapy bitterly angry and depressed. A former police officer, he had then worked as a security guard at a large industrial plant. He reported that his depression had begun three months earlier when, after leaving work one day, he was arrested for speeding and handcuffed. Sam became highly irate when the arresting officers were rude to him. The more Sam protested that he had not been speeding and questioned their procedure, stating that he knew that they were not following protocol because he had been a police officer himself, the more forceful the officers became. Sam ended up at the police station on charges of speeding and resisting arrest.

Sam became so upset that he couldn't return to work and was given a leave of absence. When his court case was heard, Sam was ordered to therapy. At the first appointment, he blamed his current state on the events of three months earlier, indicating that he desperately wanted to get back to work and resume his normal functioning. Sam reported that prior to his arrest, he had had an active social life, but since the incident, he refused to answer the telephone and spent his time watching television, sleeping, and ruminating over the episode with the police officers.

Sam stated that he lived on a large piece of property that was being overrun by weeds because of his inactivity. It was suggested that he spend four hours a day working in his garden. During that time, Sam was to remind himself that he was there because of the incident with the police officers—that he was in the garden working for them instead of being at his job. Two weeks later, Sam returned to therapy and reported that he had effectively "weeded" the anger out of his system. He realized that the police officers needed to be punished, but that he was the only one suffering. He returned to work, and also filed a complaint with their superior about the officers' rudeness.

In the preceding case, an external event penetrated to the interior. Once it was restored to the outside, a resolution was achieved. In many situations, there is a continual interplay between the external event and internal functioning, and treatment needs to address the origin of the problem and the likely means of restoring balance.

Consider the analogy of what happens when a person is shot, a situation in which an external stimulus penetrates the body's defensive systems and enters the interior. In some cases, if the individual is healthy and the bullet is accessible, surgery can be performed at once to remove it. Other situations are more complicated. If the person is frail, having lost a lot of blood, or is suffering from other medical complications, surgery may be deferred until he or she is strong enough to handle it. Similarly, if the bullet is lodged in an inaccessible location, the decision may be made to leave it alone, allowing the body to develop a protective shield around the object, isolating it from other systems. This is effective, unless the defenses around the bullet deteriorate, and the metal begins to poison the rest of the body. At that time, the person must be strengthened as much as possible so the bullet can be removed.

Treatment protocols work in a similar manner in the Eastern system. If an external influence manages to penetrate to the interior of the body, treatment can be directed toward either pulling it back to the outside or strengthening the interior to handle the trauma, depending on the nature of the pathogen and the relative health of the client. At times, the internal event can be walled off, isolating it from the rest of the system in an inert state. If this dissociative strategy fails and the body begins to become affected by the intrusion, efforts must be made to pull the problem to the exterior. Treatment strategies for handling external events that penetrate to the interior can be summarized as:

1. If possible, when the external event first occurs, strengthen the antipathogenic *qi* and pull the influence to the outside. (Ascertain that the person is strong enough to allow the bullet to be removed right away.)
2. If the pathogen reaches the interior and disrupts functioning, work to balance and promote the healthy functioning of the internal system. (Leave the bullet alone until you can strengthen the individual.)
3. If the external event penetrates to the interior and the individual manages to isolate it so that it doesn't affect other systems, leave it alone and promote the general well-being of the client. (Leave the bullet alone and address other areas of weakness unrelated to the shooting.)
4. If the protective shell begins to deteriorate, strengthen the other systems as much as possible and draw the problem to the outside. (Prepare the person as well as you can so that the bullet can be removed.)

These strategies have enormous implications for psychotherapy. First, they suggest that the best treatment for an acute traumatic episode is to strengthen the person's defense and support systems and disperse the event to the outside as soon as possible. For instance, if someone has been sexually assaulted, therapy could help to restore the person's patterns of eating and sleeping, provide relaxation strategies, and assist in developing plans to make the client feel safe and supported. The goal would be to acknowledge the client's trauma, while strengthening the person's resources and normalizing life as quickly as possible, keeping the assault in the perspective of an event external to the client as an individual.

If these strategies are unsuccessful, owing either to the enormity of the event or to the poor coping strengths of the individual, and the trauma becomes internalized, efforts should be made to strengthen other existing systems and relationships to help cope with the problem. Positive interactions with the family might be promoted or other personal resources could be called upon to help restore healthy functioning.

In situations in which a sexual assault has been completely repressed and the person has dissociated from the event, the problem need not be addressed unless or until it begins to affect other areas of functioning. Many people successfully repress events that happened in their childhood, using their dissociation as an adaptive strategy for isolating material with which it is too difficult to cope. Their defense mechanisms allow them to function in the world by keeping disruptive and paralyzing information away from awareness. The repressed memory only becomes a problem when the protective barrier is too weak to keep the event from affecting the system, in the same manner that a bullet ceases to be isolated from the body and begins to be toxic. If the individual has difficulty establishing relationships, starts to hallucinate, or develops sleep disruptions, strategies should be considered to bring the trauma into the external domain so that it can be addressed. Before this is accomplished, however, the individual's personal and interpersonal resources should be strengthened and corroboration of the trauma ascertained. To continue the metaphor, a therapist who implants or implies false memories based on the appearance of likely symptoms would be guilty of shooting the client!

Schools of therapy differ in how similar they are to the Eastern approach. For many psychodynamic systems, any repression is harmful. People are encouraged to explore every aspect of an event to ensure that they do not carry it with them. As mentioned earlier, the elaborate processing of an occurrence can make it larger than life, and too enormous for the individual to defend against. In the same way, dragging information out of isolation can often disrupt systems that are intact or totally unbalance fragile functioning. Psychodynamic therapies also do not succeed in drawing the internal event out of the individual. It is externalized in the sense that it is brought from the unconscious domain into the level of conscious processing, but the insight often doesn't make the final transition into action and resolution.

## Relational Dichotomies

The problem of an internal/external dichotomy has received considerable attention in psychotherapy. Heredity/environment, conscious/unconscious, internal locus of control/external locus of control, intrapersonal/interpersonal are all attempts to divide the world into internal and external components. The formation of an internal and external dichotomy, however, can be no more fixed than its parent categorization of *yin* and *yang*. The relationship between internal and external is constantly fluctuating, rather than being a concrete division into component parts, and the separation is certainly not placed at the skin barrier.

In Eastern terms, dichotomies are not absolute, but are relative. The question always has to be asked: "In relation to what?" A phobic thought might be more external than a vague apprehension but more internal than running away from a feared object, in the same way that muscles are interior to skin but external in relation to the organs. Nothing is by definition either internal or external; it only has that quality in comparison with something else.

In the original analytic sense, an individual was divided into conscious (external) and unconscious (internal) levels. One often reflected the other, and, as in Eastern healing, events in the interior of the psyche were considered more profound and significant than was external behavior. Therapy was directed toward uncovering the internal world and making it more accessible. The goal of many psychodynamic approaches was to free repression, bringing events and feelings to the external level where they could be observed and handled.

The division between internal and external components within the system, however, is not as fixed as might be supposed. If one considers various reflections of the unconscious, for example, a more relational view is obtained. Repressed memories are more internal than dreams, which are more internal than thoughts, which are more internal than slips of the tongue. Each is more externally oriented and articulated than the previous one, although all would be considered internal when compared with direct action.

As therapy developed, some systems rebelled against the notion of a hidden, internal psyche, questioning its existence, or at least its relevance. Behaviorists preferred to focus on a more observable, external world. Rational-emotive and cognitive therapists also followed the trend toward the external by adding a behavioral reframing. Even purely behavioral therapy systems, however, had both internal and external components. Reinforcement schedules (external) operated in the context of an organism that also had internal processes, such as reward histories and motivational drive levels.

Issues subsequently shifted to whether therapy should consider events on an intrapersonal (internal) level or focus on interpersonal (external) systems. In comparison with intrapersonal therapy, a systems approach is external. The former concentrates on events within an individual and the latter on outside interactions. Either system, however, has both internal and external components.

Intrapersonal therapy focuses on internal processes, but observes them in the context of external behaviors. If a patient discusses feelings, reports a dream, or lets out a primal scream, that patient has taken an internal event and made it external. In a hypnotic induction, there are continual interplay and fluctuations between the unconscious and conscious, the internal and external. The hypnotist (external) induces a shift in state (external to internal) in the subject. A suggestion (external) to the unconscious mind of the subject (internal) is expected to operate in such a way as to alter future perceptions (internal) and behavior (external). It is as if the hypnotist has introduced a magic bullet into the unconscious of the subject, which diffuses not toxic particles, but possibilities, into both the conscious and unconscious mind.

Even in interpersonal approaches, such as family therapy, there are relative differences in how internally or externally the system operates.

Structural therapy focuses on interpersonal relationships (external), but within the context of the family constellation (internal). To effect change within the system, one has to alter the structure of the family dynamics, not just its interplay. Strategic therapy is relatively more external than structural therapy, but such concepts as metaphor and the addressing of underlying issues have strong internal components.

Eastern philosophy encourages us to look beyond the artificial dichotomies formed by the skin and the senses. In a relational sense, internal and external components are necessarily both present, in the same way that one cannot have *yin* except in relation to *yang*. The concepts are most useful as a model for comparison and a suggestion for treatment.

# CHAPTER FIVE

## Heat and Cold

■

*Movement overcomes cold.*
*Stillness overcomes heat.*
*Stillness and tranquillity set things in*
*order in the universe.*

*—Lao-tzu*

*The brook wanders through the valley. It sparkles and splashes over rocks, cascading and rolling its way downstream. Leaves fall into the water, and their reds and yellows dance to the water's song. As autumn gives way to winter, the air chills and frost forms. Soon the cold sets in. The brook slows and then stops, leaves frozen in their flight.*

*The pot of water sits on the stove. As it heats, bubbles form and rise, pushing their way to the top. As the heat intensifies, the water begins to roll and churn. Steam surges upward and outward. Agitated, the water boils, spilling out of its container. As the heat continues, all of the water evaporates, finally cracking the container.*

These two images of water demonstrate the effects of heat and cold, another pair of the eight principles. Heat and cold detail the nature of a problem, its direction of movement, and its capacity for change. The pair can be taken both metaphorically and directly. Hot conditions feel hot to the touch and often seem too hot to handle; cold disorders can chill you to the bone.

Heat and cold produce very different reactions in nature, the body, and the spirit. The two primary results of cold are contraction and stagnation. Generally, the colder something becomes, the less movement there is. If something becomes cold enough, movement ceases altogether. Cold also produces contraction and shrinkage (just ask any male who has jumped into an icy pool!). Ice cubes in a tray have a smaller volume than when they were liquid.

Heat causes the opposite response and creates expansion and upward movement. Hot-air balloons rise as the air inside becomes warm; tissues swell with the application of heat. Adding warmth stimulates motion, but if the heat is too intense, the movement becomes agitated and difficult to contain.

## Diagnosis

### *Cold*

In Eastern healing, one diagnoses a cold disorder when the client feels cold to the touch, the pulse is slow, the tongue and face are pale, and the person's problems are ameliorated by the application of warmth. Cold causes both *qi* and *xue* to slow and stop. Masses, such as cysts and tumors, can form because movement is insufficient to disperse stagnation.

Similar problems are evident on an emotional level. Individuals with cold disorders can have icy demeanors, a tendency to stagnation, and difficulty in reacting interpersonally. Problems involving lack of affect, sexual frigidity, anorexia, impotence, depression, enuresis, and narcissism can be linked to a predominance of cold in the system. Intrapersonal therapy with these clients proceeds slowly because they are withdrawn and unable to move on issues; interpersonal therapy is marked by a distancing or isolation of the participants and slow progress.

Katie, a 35-year-old physical therapist, came to therapy complaining that her husband, Tim, rarely had sex with her and never discussed his feelings. If Tim moved off the couch at all, it was to do something in isolation and never with her. Katie said that Tim had never been very demonstrative, but since losing his job as the manager of a small engineering firm two years previously, his advances had decreased seriously. Tim didn't seem to want contact with her, or with anyone else for that matter. Katie said that any attempts to be supportive resulted in Tim's withdrawing further. When she made sexual advances, Tim would wrap himself in the bed sheets. Even when she approached him for help in deciding whether or not to accept a promotion to head of her unit at work, Katie came up against a brick wall.

Katie felt she was the only active participant in their relationship—generating most of their income, fostering connection between them, and making advances. Katie said she was known as the "ice maiden" at work. Although viewed as fair and competent, no one could accuse her of exuding warmth or giving compliments freely. Her attitude created some difficulty with her staff and formed the basis of her reluctance to accept a promotion. It was ironic to Katie that while she was considered cold and unfeeling at work, at home she was the only warm body around.

### *Heat*

Heat causes a reaction opposite to that of cold in that it creates warmth, expansion, and movement. At beneficial levels, heat promotes growth, development, and the free circulation of *qi* and *xue*. When heat levels become too high, the blood boils, the energy rises, and the body dries out. In Eastern healing, a heat disorder can be diagnosed when any of the following symptoms are present: a hot or feverish body, red face or eyes, a rapid pulse, a red or furrowed tongue, dry tissues, or hemorrhage.

On an emotional level, the rising and expanding properties of heat can cause violent outbursts of temper, mania, restlessness, agitation, and irritability. "Hot" clients can often be resistant, hostile, or reactive. Family therapy exchanges are heated, with a high level of verbal output and frequent interruptions. Fires seem to rage within and among participants, and sessions are marked by action. Change is often rapid, but unstable.

Jermaine, age 15, was sent to therapy by the group home where he lived. The referral indicated that his behavior was violent and volatile, and that he was defiant of authority. Jermaine's mother had died when he was 10, the result of a drive-by shooting. His father was an alcoholic who cared about his son, but was generally unreliable when he was drinking. Jermaine and his two sisters were first sent to live with an elderly grandmother who was in poor health, and this was followed by a stay with an uncle who physically abused him. Jermaine came to the group home at the age of 14. His behavior was difficult from the time of his arrival, but deteriorated even further because of his close friendship with another boy, William, who was placed in the home after he had attempted to murder his parents. William liked to get into trouble whenever he was bored and encouraged Jermaine to act tough. Jermaine was abrasive and argumentative when he arrived for therapy. He refused to sit in a chair and spent his time pacing around the room, hurling profanities at the therapist and kicking furniture. His attention was rarely focused, except when he was examining the stereo equipment on the shelf.

As with the other principles discussed so far, the dichotomy of heat and cold should be seen as relative rather than fixed. A problem or individual can be perceived as hot or cold, but in relation to what? An angry retort is hot in relation to an analytical comment, but colder than a violent outburst. Katie was cold in relation to her coworkers but warm in relation to her husband. Any characteristic should be considered in its current and historical context, as well as where it fits into the general pattern.

Heat and cold, like *yin* and *yang*, are transformational in addition to being relative. One can often transform into the other, especially when peak levels are reached. At the apex of a fever, a patient can suddenly become chilled and cold to the touch. Bipolar fluctuations often involve a radical shift from mania to depressive behavior at the height of an episode. As discussed in *The Art of Using and Losing Control* (Whiteside, 1998), exaggerating the presenting problem of a hostile client often forces a transition to a more complacent state.

Transformations of heat and cold can occur both intrapersonally and interpersonally. An individual might withdraw from his or her spouse and then lash out at the spouse. Similarly, the intense cold of one family member might create a hot reaction in another.

Amanda, 16, and her mother, Gertie, came to therapy after Amanda had overdosed on aspirin. Gertie had divorced Amanda's father, Peter, when the girl was three years old. The mother and daughter had been close and supportive, but Peter kept himself detached from the pair. On her 15th birthday, Amanda received a present from her father and a note saying that he wanted to reenter her life. Amanda was elated and welcomed her father's new role. Gertie resented Peter's sudden desire to be part of their lives again and suspected his motives.

Whenever Amanda would return excited from a visit with her father, Gertie would become cold and withdrawn. She accused her daughter of loving her father more than herself and suggested that she might be happier living with him. Despite Amanda's protests that no one could take her mother's special place in her heart, Gertie remained unyielding. She often would not speak to Amanda for days after her paternal visits. Eventually, Amanda would become hysterical, breaking through Gertie's defenses. This pattern recurred after every visit, until, finally, Amanda reacted by taking the overdose of aspirin.

In this case, an intensely cold posture created a hot reaction. Members of a social unit can also cycle in unison through the hot and cold transformations. The climate of the family shifts as the conditions change.

Marta arrived at the Women's Refuge after being beaten by her husband, Mel. Marta, a 24-year-old receptionist, had endured physical violence for much of her five-year marriage to Mel. She had been to the refuge twice before, and this time she was determined to leave her husband for good. When asked what was different, Marta said that she was now worried that the violence would be directed to her two small children.

Marta stated that each time violence occurred, it followed the same pattern. Mel would ignore Marta, barely speaking to her or acknowledging her presence. She would respond in kind, usually resenting him for his treatment or her last beating. Eventually, things would shift. Marta would become irritable because of her being made responsible for the care of the home and the children; Mel would be surly because of his job. Eventually, their disagreements would escalate into a screaming argument, and Mel would become violent. After the fight, Marta would be cold and detached, and Mel would withdraw from the family. The pattern would repeat until Marta got sufficiently upset to retreat to the refuge.

Therapy used the grandparents and Marta's concern for her children to disrupt the cycle. Both sets of grandparents threatened to take the children away from Mel and Marta if they didn't stop the violent episodes. All four grandparents rotated through the role of observer, defusing the situation if they suspected it was getting out of hand. One of the grandmothers was particularly adept at cajoling the couple out of their detachment and a grandfather was able to stifle Mel's aggression. The violence in the family decreased significantly. Marta eventually moved out of the relationship, however, taking the children with her. She said that she was unable to forget Mel's behavior toward her and preferred to live away from him. The couple arranged to share parental responsibilities.

The transformation of heat into cold takes place developmentally as well. In Eastern medicine, children are described as "hot diseases" because they have very rapid pulses, run around a lot, and have a great deal of energy and labile emotional responses. With age, however, there is a decrease in the *yang* heat available. Adults tend to be more sedentary than children and cooler in their appraisals. With the advent of old age, the heat declines even further, leaving the elderly person sensitive to cold drafts and encumbered by stiff joints.

## Treatment

Treatment protocols are generally straightforward in relation to heat and cold: if something is too cold, warm it up; if it is too hot, cool it down. The exception is when one chooses to exaggerate the properties, pushing heat and cold to such extreme limits that they transform. As with most therapy techniques, one usually is better off trying a less intrusive intervention first, and turning to more radical strategies if the initial attempts are unsuccessful.

### *Cold*

Because cold causes contraction and stagnation, treatment principles should be directed toward creating movement and expansion. This could take the form of exercise, suggestions for action, or connecting people in an interpersonal sense. The intensity of cold and its level determine how quickly therapy can proceed. If an individual is frozen, it takes more energy and warmth to create a thaw than if the person is merely chilled.

While Katie was describing her frustration with Tim and his lack of sexual interest, Tim would seem to withdraw from the room, his eyes glazing over and his interest diminishing. When asked to comment or participate, Tim would shrug and indicate that he didn't have much to add. Any suggestions were met with a noncommittal response or weak agreement. Katie finally lashed out, stating that if Tim wouldn't agree to intensify their relationship, she would find sexual fulfillment elsewhere. She said that she didn't feel that she could leave him, but she wanted her needs met by someone. Katie's outburst created a slight shift in Tim's demeanor. He said that he wanted their marriage to continue, and he certainly didn't want her sleeping with another man. When the therapist asked Katie what a minimum level of sexual interaction would be for her, she said that she would feel satisfied if they were intimate twice a week. Tim was placed in charge of initiating sexual contact at least two times a week to ensure his more active role in the relationship. As therapy continued, the couple reported an increase in warmth in their interactions to an acceptable, if not passionate, level.

***Heat***

Heat causes motion, primarily in an upward and outward direction. Treatment protocols for hot conditions should stress cooling things down and increasing stability. Individuals in a high state of heat agitation react with volatility to any suggestion. Attempts must be made to decrease motility and increase a sense of calm. Since the movement of heat is essentially outward and upward, any intervention that contains action within a person or redirects it to a more appropriate target is beneficial.

Jermaine's hostility in therapy was tempered somewhat by a degree of remorse about his delinquent actions and a positive connection with some of the staff members at the group home. Therapy consisted of gradually separating him from William, both at the home and in school. This was most easily achieved by stimulating Jermaine's interest in electronic equipment. Therapy sessions were able to be conducted with Jermaine in a seated position as long as he could tinker with the office's broken heater or cassette recorder while he talked. An after-school job in a repair shop was arranged, and the shop's owner became so impressed with Jermaine's talent that he would invite him home to dinner. Jermaine became a frequent visitor, eventually allowing the family's warmth and concern to temper his hostility.

## In Conclusion

The relationship of heat and cold is both oppositional and complementary, affecting aspects of warmth and movement. Understanding the relationship between the two principles facilitates both the diagnosis and the development of treatment strategies. The interplay between heat and cold and the other six principles is considered in Chapter 7.

# CHAPTER SIX

## Excess and Deficiency

■

*For one gains by losing*
*And loses by gaining.*

—*Lao-tzu*

*The stream flows between its banks, oblivious to the storm raging around it. A sharp crack, and a tree struck by lightning falls across the water. Gradually, debris and pools of water begin to accumulate upstream from the fallen tree. On the downstream side of the obstacle, only a trickle of water can squeeze past. If the tree continues to obstruct the flow, over time the pools of water upstream will become stagnant and rank, and the area below the fallen tree, parched and desolate.*

For nature or the body to remain healthy, there should be a constant flow of adequate energy. The principles of excess and deficiency describe the consequences that result when there is either too much or too little of a required substance. Like all of the other principles, there is no absolute or static level of sufficiency. Requirements fluctuate in relation to environmental events and individual characteristics, in much the same way that a woman's nutritional needs would differ depending on whether she was a teenager, was pregnant, or was postmenopausal.

Deficiency literally is having too little of something, whether it's *qi*, *xue*, or attention; excess, conversely, results when there is too much of a particular substance. The factors can occur in relation to each other or independently. For example, a person might be very "normal," but an excess of stress at work will cause a breakdown in functioning. Similarly, another person might have insufficient interpersonal contact or affection, although the rest of the person's life is on course

Like the tree in the example, many stressful life events can create obstructions in intrapersonal or interpersonal functioning. The block often results in a buildup of frustration and an inability to move in a productive direction.

> Marcia and Tony had been married for five years. They wanted desperately to buy a home of their own, but it seemed that every time they accumulated enough funds for a down payment, an emergency would arise that would frustrate their plan and decrease their savings. Despite previous setbacks, Marcia and Tony had once again gathered enough money to make the down payment on a small house. Two days before they were to sign the papers for the sale, Tony had an automobile accident that totaled his vehicle. Marcia lashed out at him, screaming at his stupidity and continual destruction of their lives. Tony withdrew in a sulk, refusing to go to work or to talk with his wife.

The car accident in this example worked much like the tree across the stream. The event obstructed the flow of the couple's plan, resulting in an excess of anger on Marcia's part and a deficiency of energy and action on Tony's.

The concepts of deficiency and excess have relevance to therapy with regard to both diagnosis and treatment. By understanding a client in relation to these principles, a therapist can direct the therapy toward more successful resolution.

## Deficiency

Basically, anything in the system can become depleted and result in a deficiency. Increased demands within or outside of an individual use up available resources, and without compensation, a shortage develops. Similarly, the balance within a person can be fine, but outside events can occur (food shortages, the death of a loved one, rejection by a partner) that cause the input of a necessary substance to fall below acceptable levels. The resulting scarcity of food, comfort, or love can create a deficiency in the client. In Eastern healing, the two most common types of insufficiencies are *qi* and *xue* deficiencies.

### *Qi Deficiency*

*Qi* deficiencies can be caused by improper diet, old age, or constitutional weakness. Continual overwork or chronic stress can also consume *qi* and result in insufficient levels of energy. Deficient-*qi* clients present as listless and feeble. They often dislike speaking because it takes too much energy, and if they do talk, their voices are low and breathless. These clients frequently sit slumped in a chair, with a lethargic demeanor, showing little or no interest in external events. Action seems beyond them, and physical or mental exertion tends to make the situation worse. Energy levels are often too low to fulfill *qi*'s function of holding things in their place, so there can be sweating for no reason or leakage of urine or sperm.

> Steve, a 22-year-old who lived in a group home, appeared for therapy. He looked almost emaciated, with a pale face and dark circles under his eyes. Steve had lived in a series of facilities since leaving his family home at the age of 17, when he was hospitalized for being delusional. He had no friends and depended on the mental health system to meet his basic needs. Steve often would stare vaguely at the therapist when asked a direct question, and would sigh rather than give an answer. The group home was anxious that Steve find some employment or interests.

Interventions that demand action usually fail with a client who is deficient in *qi*, because they require the person to use energy that he or she doesn't have. Therapists often become frustrated with deficient-*qi* clients because they won't make the slightest effort, even to do things that would probably make them feel better. Compliance, however, requires *qi*. A client who does not have enough energy either cannot act or will burn up vital source *qi* in trying to cooperate. This usually leaves the person more deficient at the end of the intervention than before the attempt. For therapy to be successful with deficient-*qi* clients, energy must be provided from an outside source.

Steve's family was brought into therapy with him. He was overwhelmed by the fact that his parents cared enough to attend sessions and admitted that he felt his constant institutionalization had been caused by their unwillingness to love him. Treatment focused on having Steve's parents demonstrate through actions how much they cared for him. Eventually, the therapy linked the family's efforts and interest to stimulating productive initiatives in Steve.

### *Xue* Deficiency

A depletion of *xue* can be caused by insufficient food intake, excessive blood loss, or drastic emotional changes. Individuals with a *xue* deficiency often have sallow complexions and pale lips. Because the blood is not performing its nourishing function adequately, there frequently is blurring of vision, a vague dizziness, memory loss, insomnia, and weakness or numbness in the limbs.

The delivery of her third child had taken its toll on Clara. Labor had lasted 32 hours, and she had hemorrhaged toward the end. She didn't feel like caring for the baby, and even if the infant slept through the night, Clara didn't. Her mouth felt dry all the time, her scalp was flaking and her hair was limp, and her legs ached with a dull throb. Every time she tried to force herself to get moving, she felt even worse.

As in *qi* deficiencies, a deficiency of *xue* requires some sort of supplementation as treatment. The body has to be nourished and rested so that levels can return to normal. Additionally, because *qi* and *xue* are closely related, a deficiency of one can result in a depletion of the other, with the client's presenting symptoms of both. Treatment in these cases would need to provide both succor and energy to ensure recovery.

## Excess

Excesses occur when too much of something is present in the system. This could be attributable to extremely high levels of food intake, stress, disease, or emotion. Excesses can also be generated within the body. While there is unlikely to be an overabundance of some functions or substances (*jing* or *shen*, for instance), there can be a problem if too much *qi* or *xue* accumulates. The excess is caused by a cessation of flow, resulting in too much energy or blood pooling in one place. The situation is similar to that of the water that was dammed up by the fallen tree. If water, or *qi*, or *xue* is not allowed to flow and circulate, it stagnates and causes problems.

### *Stagnation of Qi*

The circulation of energy in the body can become obstructed by mental agitation or depression, a diet rich in fatty or cold foods, or the invasion of an external pathogen (wind, cold, heat, etc.). The onset of symptoms is often linked to eating, emotional stimuli, or external events. *Qi* stagnation may be marked by pain and swelling, such as the distention of abdomen and breasts seen premenstrually or the discomfort of a sprained ankle. Distention takes place because energy and fluids aren't moving past obstructions in the system, and so begin to accumulate and pool. Symptoms appear and disappear sporadically, as energy manages to break through the blockage at some times, but not at others. Irritability, swings in emotion, and uneven reactions can be indicative of an excess caused by *qi* stagnation.

Frustration is a good example of *qi* obstruction. By definition, frustration arises when a goal or desire cannot be fulfilled. Thwarting effort creates a block to action, and stops the flow from intent to achievement. This obstruction creates a number of emotional responses, all of which would be classified as excess in nature.

Treatment for *qi* stagnation involves removing the cause of the blockage and restoring smooth flow, as in lifting the tree from the path of the stream. If the obstruction has been severe, flow must be restored slowly and gradually, so that flooding doesn't result when the block is removed. In cases where an obstruction can't be eliminated, a detour must be created that allows for free flow around the problem.

Chuck presented for therapy as an overworked, burned-out, business executive charged with the task of downsizing a major corporation. On good days, he went to work at 7 A.M. and didn't get home until midnight; on bad days, he slept in his office. Chuck's wife, Katrina, was generally understanding, but lately, she and their 15-year-old daughter had become concerned about his behavior. Chuck experienced wide fluctuations of emotion. He was irritated most of the time, becoming deeply distressed over the destruction of a company that he had helped build and desperately sad about the number of valuable employees he would have to let go. Chuck knew that he was stressed out, but he couldn't see a way out of the situation. Therapy centered on getting Chuck to set priorities and delegate responsibility, relieving the pressure he was experiencing. Gradually, he was able to bring his work back to a more manageable level.

#### *Stagnation of Xue*

Blood can accumulate as the result of sprains, contusions, poor *qi* circulation, or an excess of cold in the system. *Xue* stagnation is marked by pain that is fixed and stabbing, the possible accumulation of masses or tumors, and purplish marks on the skin or tongue. A high level of pain during menstruation, accompanied by clotting in the discharge, is symptomatic of *xue* stagnation. Generally, treatment for *xue* stagnation is similar to that for *qi* stagnation—remove the cause of the blockage and restore smooth flow.

Excess states do not respond well to the addition of more energy. The condition is already full of energy, so increasing pressure could make it explode. Clients who have problems of an excess nature sometimes present as resistant or oppositional, since the "fullness" of their situation precludes their taking in additional suggestions or input. In line with the adjustments suggested by transpositional therapy (Whiteside, 1998), clients who give a therapist no control do much better when therapy is redirected to topics that are not as volatile. This happens because the client is able to receive input regarding an area that is not in excess, even if he or she is not open to suggestions about an issue that is "full."

### Combinations of Deficiency and Excess

Variations of excesses and deficiencies can exist both intrapersonally and interpersonally. An individual can be overworked and underloved. One member of a family might be violent and aggressive while another is depressed and lethargic. In Eastern healing, treatment focuses on balancing the system, using the surplus of the excess condition to feed the weakness of the deficiency. This strategy can also be applied to therapy.

There are times when a client will obsess about one part of his or her life, ignoring other facets until they shrink to insignificance. A woman who concentrates exclusively on her career and never on her children, a man who flaunts his sexuality and loses his compassion, and a teenager who hangs out with friends and forgets the family are all examples of concurrent excesses and deficiencies. In each of these cases, treatment needs to address the imbalance and restore more harmonious functioning by channeling the excess into a more deficient area.

> Jimmy, a 14-year-old boy, came to therapy because of an obsession with cleanliness. He had difficulty maintaining friendships because he berated others for their slovenliness. He had come to live with his mother, Nancy, after a five-year stay with a violent father. Things had started out fine, but recently Jimmy had begun to hit Nancy whenever she suggested that the house was clean enough. Nancy said she loved Jimmy and wanted to keep him with her. Although the police were frequently called during her son's outbursts, she never pressed charges.
>
> It was decided to use Jimmy's "excess" levels of cleaning activity and aggressive behavior to address his "deficient" peer relationships. He agreed to attend classes at a local karate school. The school stressed traditional values of self-discipline and personal responsibility, applying them to the appropriate use of violence and care of personal space. Jimmy happily helped to clean the facility before and after class. The other students often chose Jimmy as a partner for work details because he received such high praise from the teacher. He was also well regarded because of his exceptional skills in karate. Jimmy accepted the school's rule of "no violence" outside of class, except in self-defense. As he spent more time at the school and with friends from the class, he paid less attention to his mother's care of their home and was more accepting of her appraisal of their house as being sufficiently clean.

Concurrent deficiencies and excesses can exist on an interpersonal level as well. Couples often present as incompatible when the energy levels of one partner are at odds with those of the other. The depressive, lethargic behavior of one family member might frustrate another, leading to a state of excessive irritation and agitation.

Clyde, a 53-year-old sales executive, lost his job when his company was bought by a conglomerate. He was given a large severance payment, but despaired of finding another position before his funds ran out. He spent most days sitting at home, watching business programs and soap operas on television, and rarely making it out of his pajamas. He didn't have much appetite and wasn't sleeping well. When his grandchildren came for a visit, he generally ignored them or sent them to another room because they annoyed him. His wife of 28 years, Carol, was becoming very upset with the situation. Carol had never worked, but prided herself on the energy and commitment she devoted to her family and community projects. Her whole routine was disrupted by Clyde's inactivity. She couldn't stand his laziness and slovenliness and considered his presence and his need for her attention extremely inconvenient. The more Carol berated Clyde, the more lethargic he became.

Therapy sought to address the imbalance between the couple. Initial attempts centered on trying to get Clyde more involved with projects while reducing Carol's participation, but Clyde never carried out agreed-upon tasks, which led to increased irritation on the part of his wife. The therapist felt that if Clyde wanted to sit, he might as well do it in a way that would benefit him. The couple had always been religious, and so arrangements were made for Clyde to attend a religious retreat in the mountains. For two weeks, he could sit and contemplate his situation, but in a more acceptable setting. Carol would have two weeks during which she could attend to her projects without Clyde's interference.

Clyde returned from the retreat with renewed vigor and enthusiasm. He said that he had reconnected with his spiritual self, and the piety and devotion of the brothers had been inspirational. He applied himself to looking for work and filled the empty spaces by participating in church projects rather than watching television. Carol had relaxed considerably during this time away and appreciated the change in Clyde. She was able to establish a comfortable schedule for working on her projects and spending time with her family, as Clyde was taking care of himself and often was out looking for work or at church. Sometimes, the couple also participated in joint community ventures.

## In Conclusion

The principle of excess and deficiency helps therapists understand the quality of a problem by observing whether there is too much or too little of something present. By defining a situation as excess or deficient, a suitable treatment strategy can be selected to restore interpersonal or intrapersonal balance.

# CHAPTER SEVEN

## The Eight Principles and Differential Diagnosis

■

*The Tao of heaven is like the bending of a*
*bow.*
*The high is lowered and the low is raised.*
*If the string is too long, it is shortened;*
*If there is not enough, it is made longer.*

*—Lao-tzu*

The preceding chapters described the eight principles—*yin/yang*, cold/heat, internal/external, deficiency/excess—and showed ways in which they might be useful in psychotherapy. In Eastern healing, the eight principles form the foundation of differential diagnosis. Each case is evaluated in terms of the dichotomous pairs so that an appropriate treatment plan can be developed. Differential diagnosis based on the model defines a condition in relation to all of the features simultaneously. *Yin* and *yang* are the overriding principles, in that cold, deficiency, and internal are all *yin* qualities, and heat, excess, and external are all *yang* features. (See Table 7.1.)

| *YIN* | *YANG* |
|---|---|
| Cold | Heat |
| Internal | External |
| Deficiency | Excess |

**Table 7.1.** *The Eight Principles*

■

Although the overall nature of a condition can be *yin* or *yang*, it is more accurately described as a combination of several principles; that is, as external, cold, and excess or internal, hot, and deficient. The principles can combine in any permutation, and, at times, two very different patterns can be present simultaneously in an individual. For example, if a weak, elderly person with an internal configuration of *qi* and heat deficiency were to catch pneumonia (an external, hot, excess problem), symptoms of all eight principles would be present at the same time. The same complex patterns can arise in therapy situations.

> Toni presented for therapy after witnessing her daughter being run over by a car on the street outside of her home. The girl's injuries were minor and her recovery complete, but Toni is not handling the matter well. She can't sleep without dreaming of the accident, and her mind races constantly. Toni becomes hysterical at random times during the day. She blames the accident on her own inability to care for her daughter properly. Toni said she had been despondent and depressed for the past year. She is listless and eats poorly. Her lack of energy was the reason that she had monitored her daughter's activities from her window instead of going with her into the yard.

Toni's chronic internal deficiencies are present at the same time as her acute external excess reactions, creating difficulty in coping with the stressful event and prolonging her recovery. Her reactions and ability to heal would be different from those of a person with strong antipathogenic *qi* in similar circumstances, because symptoms of deficiency would not be present in the pattern.

Any case, then, can be differentiated by where it sits in relation to each of the eight principles at a specific time. Understanding the interrelation of the pairs allows for the formulation of a treatment plan to restore balance and promote healthy functioning. The advantage of a dichotomous system, such as the eight principles, is that it generally indicates the direction of treatment. If a person is too hot, make him or her colder; if something is deficient, increase it; if a problem is internal, externalize it. While this results in a practical view toward problems, in Eastern healing, as in life, issues are rarely so simple. It would be nice in therapy if one could design interventions solely on the basis of dichotomous principles—if they're sad, make them happy; if they're distant, bring them closer; if they won't go to school, get them to attend. While many behavior-based, solution-focused, or strategic systems use this concept in principle, there are often other factors that affect the form of the intervention.

## True and False

In designing a treatment according to the eight principles, it is essential to ascertain whether a condition of excess or deficiency is present. This is can be more complicated than predicted. Consider the interplay between heat and cold and deficiency and excess depicted in Figure 7.1.

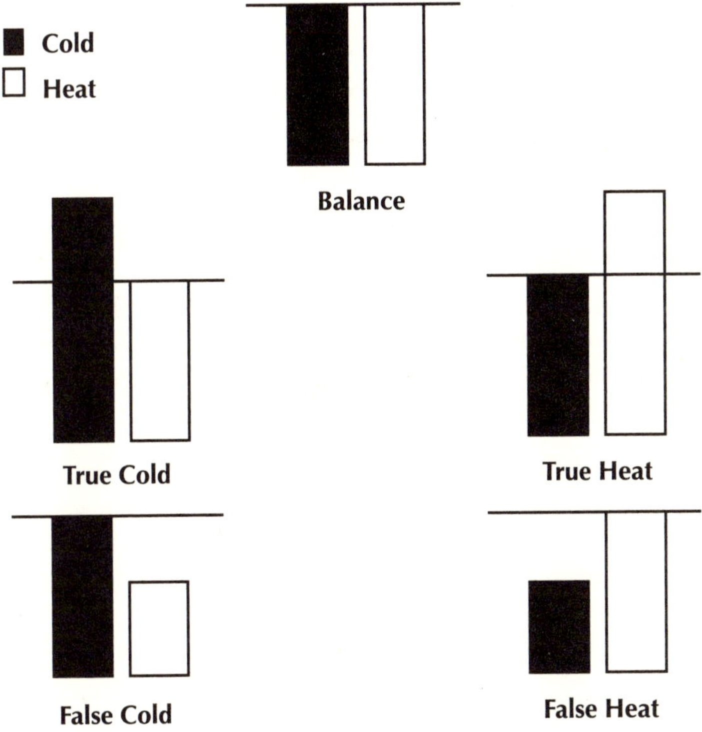


**Figure 7.1.** *Relationship of heat and cold.*

In the body, there is a "normal" level of heat and cold that should exist—the balance state. If both are present in equal and sufficient amounts, functioning will be smooth and healthy. If there is either an excess or a deficiency of one or the other, a state of imbalance is created that can produce problems. The matter becomes complicated for the diagnostician and practitioner because in both true cold, an excess situation, and false cold, a deficiency situation, the client shows similar symptoms. Since the problems stem from totally different etiologies, however, they require different courses of treatment.

In the true-cold situation, heat in the body is present at a normal level. Due to the introduction of various factors (extreme intake of raw or cold food, getting caught in an ice storm without protective clothing, constant application of ice packs), the body has acquired an overabundance of cold. True cold is an excess condition in which there are higher than normal levels of cold in the system. The first goal of treatment should be to remove the elements that produced the excess in the first place (decrease consumption of cold food or cease the application of ice packs). This diminishes the amount of cold in the system and prevents a further increase. Since cold causes contraction and stagnation, efforts must also be made to get things moving. By restoring movement and flow, the excess can be reduced to normal levels.

Adding high levels of heat is not an appropriate treatment for a true-cold condition. An excess state, by definition, already has too much of a particular substance, which, in this case, is cold. Adding energy or heat to the mix might create equilibrium, but at a point much higher than normal. While the amounts of heat and cold would be comparable, the levels of both would be extremely high. Excess situations without an accompanying deficiency require treatment that reduces rather than increases. In true-cold conditions, there is an excess of *yin* energy leading to stagnation. Increasing movement serves to decrease the overabundance of cold, removing the excess without raising the level of heat substantially.

Elaine and Jerry attended therapy for marital problems. Jerry had engaged in a series of affairs during their marriage. Elaine said that she loathed Jerry, but because of their children and her fear of a custody battle, she had suppressed her feelings. She said that they had a marriage in name only. The couple barely spoke and never had sex. If Elaine responded to Jerry at all, it was with derision and coldness. They each spent time alone with their children, rarely doing anything as a family. Their interaction, or lack of it, had stabilized over the years. The only reason the couple presented for therapy at this time was that Elaine had noticed that the children were becoming distant and moody. She worried that the couple's relationship was having a negative impact on the children's well-being. Therapy focused on the one area the couple shared: devotion to their children. Elaine and Jerry were asked to arrange mutual family outings, instilling the activities with a sense of adventure and focusing on making them as much fun as possible for their children. Gradually, as the couple interacted in the context of the family excursions, their relationship became more normal and agreeable.

Elaine and Jerry were able to reduce the level of coldness in their relationship and its resulting stagnation by creating movement in a mutually agreeable area rather than by trying to increase the warmth between them.

True-heat situations operate in a similar fashion. The body contains normal amounts of cold, but an excess of heat has entered the system (overeating hot or spicy foods, too much alcohol, suffering sunstroke, contracting a febrile disease). Treatment must reduce the levels of heat present, a process called "clearing" in Eastern healing, without significantly increasing the amount of cold. In situations of excess, the overabundance must be eliminated while maintaining the healthy levels of other factors.

Diagnosis and treatment become more complex in deficiency problems. In false-cold conditions, the system actually exhibits a normal level of cold, but its heat is insufficient. Symptoms are a product of the lack of heat rather than of the presence of excess cold. False-cold conditions require treatments different from those for true-cold problems. Diminishing the cold in this instance would further exacerbate the deficiency condition, as the individual would now be too low in both heat and cold. Since false cold is produced by a deficiency of warmth, treatment needs to add *yang* to the system, such as by increasing the level of nurturance or passion.

Harrison, a 32-year-old engineer, and his wife, Patricia, a 34-year-old attorney, came to therapy expressing a desire to improve their communication. Patricia stated that despite her best efforts, she could not get Harrison to talk to her about anything other than his work. Attempts by Patricia to get her husband to attend classes in wine tasting or to work on community projects with her were met with indifference. Harrison was content to read or watch television, but had no interest in discussing either the books or the TV shows with his wife. Their sex life was satisfactory, although not passionate, and they did socialize with friends. There just seemed to be something missing.

During therapy, Harrison revealed that no one in his family of origin had ever shown their emotions. He didn't remember his father's expressing an opinion on anything of consequence, and his mother believed that hugs created "sissies." Therapy was directed toward helping Harrison act more warmly toward Patricia and his family. Once a day, he was to do something concrete as an expression of his feelings. He could bring Patricia flowers, write a note to his mother, or help out a homeless person. The act didn't have to be big, but it had to be different from that of the day before. Harrison found it difficult at first to come up with ideas, and Patricia was allowed to help only if he asked her for assistance. By the end of the month, the couple reported a real warming of their relationship and better communication.

The situation is similar for false-heat situations. Symptoms arise because of a deficiency of cold energy, while heat is present in a normal amount. Treatment needs to restore cold to an appropriate level without reducing the degree of heat present, thus restoring balance.

The differences between true and false conditions are vital in therapy. Consider a child who has temper tantrums. A true-heat tantrum would be volatile in nature, with severe behaviors, such as head banging, screaming, and kicking. The situation would be quite "hot," with a high level of energy present. Appropriate treatment for this type of tantrum would be to reduce the excess. This could be accomplished by using "clearing" techniques, such as letting the child blow off steam in a safe and padded environment. Alternatively, the accumulation of heat could be avoided by preventing frustrating situations.

False-heat tantrums have a different quality. Deficiency conditions often differ from excess situations in the extremity of the behavior observed. Deficient problems may have the form, but not the substance, of an excess. In a false-heat tantrum, fussing and whining are more prevalent than screaming. Hitting and kicking are often accompanied by a glance at a significant person to see if that person is paying attention. False-heat situations are created by a lack of cooling, nurturing *yin* energy. Thus, treatment should concentrate on providing attention elsewhere, away from the tantrum. By giving a child nurturance when he or she is acting properly, *yin* levels increase and become more balanced with *yang*. As treatment protocols for deficiency and excess conditions differ significantly, care must be taken in the diagnostic process.

## Roots and Branches

The eight principles are critical to the development of treatment plans in Eastern healing, but there is also consideration of a problem's root and branch relationships. The root of a difficulty is similar to the concept of an underlying problem in therapy. It is the basis of disease, the primary factor causing the problem. Root issues have the longer history, having existed prior to any manifestations of the current situation. They sit at the base of a problem, feeding and supporting it, as its roots do a tree. A root system, however, depends on the soil around it and the health of the structure above. In Eastern healing, the roots are comparable to the antipathogenic *qi*, created by a continual interplay between inherent and historical events and forming the basis for interactions with environmental events in the future.

Branches can be diverse and can differ from each other, although they all spring from a common root structure. Presenting problems do not have as lengthy a history as do the underlying issues, and they often take a variety of forms. For example, the root problem of childhood sexual abuse may result in a variety of branches later in life—relationship difficulties, eating disorders, panic attacks, phobias. Because branches are more external than roots, they are often easier to access and are more easily changed. If a root structure is defective, however, no amount of pruning will save the tree. (See Table 7.2.)

| ROOT | BRANCH |
|---|---|
| Underlying problem | Presenting problem |
| Cause | Manifestation |
| Antipathogenic *qi* | Environmental factors |
| Chronic problems | Acute problems |

**Table 7.2.** *Roots and Branches.*

Historically, there have been arguments among schools of therapy as to whether treatment should focus on underlying or presenting problems. Psychodynamic approaches concentrate on the roots and regard branch aspects as trivial and superficial; behaviorist and solution-focused approaches stress presenting problems. Other treatment approaches strive to address both domains, alternating between the two.

The Eastern healing system offers insights that can help in the use of roots and branches in therapy. Before a treatment plan is formulated, an initial assessment is made of the degree of severity of the root and branch problems and their current manifestations. Serious acute problems are always given precedence. If a person is suicidal, for instance, it is probably not the time to explore underlying issues. Treatment needs to be directed toward stabilizing the situation and keeping the client safe. Once the crisis has passed, therapy can address some of the underlying difficulties that created the acute problem.

If there are no branch issues that require immediate attention, initial treatment should be directed toward underlying problems, since making the roots healthy will affect the entire system. This is particularly evident in situations in which an underlying difficulty is creating a variety of presenting problems. By addressing the root issues instead of chasing the branches, a more successful, permanent resolution can be achieved.

Jackie presented for therapy with her two children, Adam, age eight, and Ben, age three. Jackie, a 29-year-old divorced mother, said that she had become increasingly stressed over the past two years since Stan, her husband, had left her for another woman. Jackie was finding it difficult to raise her children on her own while working as a part-time clerk. She has problems with sleeping and frequent panic attacks. Jackie said that she knew that Stan had been having affairs during their marriage, but she had always felt that if she ignored them and gave him enough love, he would come back to her. But her strategy had not worked, and Stan was now living with the other woman.

The presenting problem that brought Jackie to therapy was related to Ben, who would insist on crawling all over his mother and then would bite her if she tried to stop him. During the past six months, the situation had become intolerable, with Ben increasingly finding new ways to inflict pain on his mother. Jackie had always been protective of Ben, worrying about the effect his father's leaving had had on the boy, but she said that Ben's current behavior had tested her patience to its limits.

Adam, the older son, has been having problems at school. He cannot concentrate on his work, and his grades are deteriorating. Adam becomes very anxious at home, worrying about how his mother is coping with her separation and his brother's behavior. Jackie says that Adam tries to take over Ben's discipline, and this causes fights between the two boys. During the initial session, a cycle of interaction became evident. Ben would behave in intrusive, destructive ways, and Jackie would plead with him to stop. Ben would escalate his behavior until Jackie would physically remove him, lecturing him on why he shouldn't be so clingy. Her statements would have a beneficial effect for about five minutes, at which point the cycle would start again. As the problem developed, Adam would become visibly anxious and attempt to help his mother.

Jackie said that she had grown up in a family whose members never respected each other's space. Her sisters would come into her room and take her things, but her parents refused to intervene. Her mother and father were also passive toward her sisters when they became adolescents, allowing them to stay out as late as they wished. Jackie, on the other hand, tried to be the "good kid," always obeying her parents. Therapy focused on the underlying problem of Jackie's inability to set clear boundaries with her sisters, her husband, or her children. The therapist told Jackie that each time that Ben attempted to cling to and harm her, she was to stop him without an accompanying lecture. Jackie followed these instructions and Ben became angry, but she held to her position with the support of the therapist. By the end of the session, Jackie was able not only to control Ben, but also to interest him in an independent activity on the other side of the room. During the course of therapy, Jackie became more secure in establishing boundaries. She designated specific times when Stan could visit the children instead of allowing him to disrupt their lives at random. Adam's anxiety decreased greatly, and his schoolwork and play with his brother normalized.

In this case, focusing on the root problem achieved resolution of many of the presenting difficulties. There are times, however, when the root issues are not accessible for treatment. This can happen when a client refuses to address anything but the presenting problem, denying or minimizing the underlying situation. Sometimes this stance can be attributed to the sensitivity of the core issues, as in a client who does not want to deal with traumas. Other individuals have no interest in exploring underlying issues and have come for treatment to help them with specific problems. In these cases, successfully resolving the presenting issues can create a trusting relationship between the practitioner and client that opens the door to the possible treatment of underlying problems at a later time. Additionally, because all functioning is inherently interconnected, creating a change in the presenting problem could generate improvement of underlying issues. Difficulties arise when a client's underlying problems interfere so dramatically with the presenting issues that resolution of the branch difficulties is impossible without adjustments at the roots.

An acupuncture client presented with symptoms of severe gastrointestinal pain and gas that would arise every time she ate. This had a serious impact on her ability to attend social and business lunches or dinners, since, after eating, she would double over in pain. She also had a tendency to form breast cysts and was worried about developing cancer. Interviews with the client revealed that she ate an enormous amount of chocolate every day. Despite admonitions from her doctor and gynecologist that the excessive intake of sugar and caffeine was contributing to her problems, she refused to give up her chocolate. The client maintained that she wanted help with her pain and digestion problems, but it was clear this was not going to be possible unless she adjusted the root of the difficulty.

This situation is also seen in therapy contexts. Some clients want the therapist to eliminate their presenting problems but are unwilling to make changes themselves. For therapy to be effective, the client needs to be hooked into addressing the relevant underlying issues.

Ted and Alicia came to therapy complaining that their 15-year-old daughter, Sara, refused to apply herself in school and was making failing grades. Sara had never been an outstanding student, but over the past three months, there had been a deterioration in her schoolwork and her behavior. Although she used to be bubbly and cheerful, recently her interactions with her parents were surly and negative. Both parents denied that there were other issues in the family related to Sara's problems and were anxious that the therapist "fix" their daughter. Suggestions regarding monitoring Sara's work and spending time with her in relation to her studies were met with apathy by all parties.

Problems escalated when Sara was caught skipping school and suspended for three days. Alicia and Ted were furious at Sara and began to argue violently with each other. When the therapist asked to speak with them alone, Alicia said that it didn't surprise her that Sara didn't try in school, since Ted didn't try in bed. For the past five years, Ted had shown no interest in sex and never approached his wife passionately. Alicia felt she was less of a woman since she could not interest her husband. Ted said there was no one else and he did not want to leave his family, but just had no interest in sex.

Therapy shifted to the couple's sexual problems. Ted agreed that although he had no interest in sex, it was his responsibility to please his wife sexually. He was given the role of intimacy initiator for the next two months. After that time, Ted could ask Alicia to initiate sex in a way that stimulated and pleased him. As the couple's sex life improved, Sara saw a warmer, more giving side to her parents. She began to try harder in school, eventually returning to her average level of functioning.

While a variety of symptoms might be linked to a common root, it is also true that the manifestation of similar symptoms could be produced by a variety of causes. In the medical model of diagnosis, a person is assigned a label describing his or her condition—major depression, obsessive-compulsive disorder, schizophrenia, and so on. Eastern systems also have diagnostic categories, such as "deficient spleen *qi*" or "phlegm misting the heart," for which there are traditional treatment protocols. Differential diagnosis in the Eastern system, however, requires that the components of the underlying problem and the presenting issues be specified for each individual, and that the unique qualities of the roots and branches be recognized as being as important as their commonalties. Depression, for example, could be the result of an excess or deficiency, an absence of heat or an overabundance of cold, and caused either internally or externally. What might be called by a single name in the Western system could have a wide range of causes and treatment protocols in the Eastern framework.

## In Conclusion

For differential diagnosis to result in effective treatment, there must be continual evaluation of where a problem stands in relation to the eight principles, its root cause, and its current manifestations. In the next part of this book, an additional framework is presented—the Law of Five Elements.

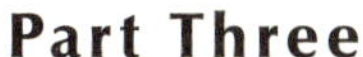

# Part Three

## THE FIVE ELEMENTS

*The five colors blind the eye.*
*The five tones deafen the ear.*
*The five flavors dull the taste*

*—Lao-tzu*

The concept of dividing the universe into primary components has existed for many thousands of years. According to ancient Oriental, Aryuvedic (Indian), and Greek healing systems, the forces of nature—the earth, air, fire, and water—existed in a patient's body and mind as a reflection and internalization of the cosmos. The elements were the foundation of both the diagnosis and the treatment of disease.

The Eastern, or Oriental, system proposed that the internal landscape can be described by five elements: Earth, Metal/Air, Water, Wood, and Fire. The essence of these natural forces was translated into constructs of physiology and behavior. The ebb and flow of environmental changes were transcribed into laws of healthy functioning. Every aspect of physical and emotional activity found a context in the structure and harmony of the universe.

In the following chapters, the characteristics of the five elements will be described and related to aspects of therapy. Finally, the Law of Five Elements—the system of growth and control between the elements—will be applied to intrapersonal and interpersonal strategies for clients.

# CHAPTER EIGHT

## Earth

■

*The valley spirit never dies;*
*It is the woman, primal mother.*

—*Lao-tzu*

The earth is our home. It provides stability and grounding. From the earth comes nourishment and the basis of fertility. Its revolutions form the cycles of our lives. It is the center and the source. Earth is substantial, solid, and slow moving. It supports us and pulls us close. The metaphor and meaning of Earth become manifest in the body, mind, and spirit. Difficulties with eating, stability, or nurturance are Earth problems. Individuals who are obsessively tied to rituals or schedules or those who can't leave home might have an imbalance in this element.

Each of the five elements is related to specific body organs. In the Eastern system, these organs are not strictly anatomical structures, but are physiological systems that serve particular functions. For this reason, the names of the organs will be captalized to discriminate them from their Western corollaries. Earth is related to the Spleen as a *yin* organ and to the Stomach as a *yang* organ. The Spleen is responsible for transportation and transformation in the body. In its transportational role, it sends fluid, food, *qi*, and *xue* to all parts of the body, nourishing the tissues and bones, keeping the mind and body functioning. If the Spleen is well, the muscles are properly formed, weight is maintained at a normal level, the mind is nourished and sound, and fluid moves freely. If there are difficulties with Spleen function and transportation is impaired, edema can result, bloating is seen, and the mind becomes stuck.

The Spleen is also in charge of transformation in both the body and spirit. On a basic level, this refers to the Spleen's role in digestion. It extracts the vital essences from food and sends them to where they belong. Poor appetite, malnutrition, or indigestion can all be related to problems in Spleen function. On a mental plane, the Spleen creates the transformation of thoughts, preventing them from becoming stuck or obsessive. Individuals with Spleen imbalances ruminate excessively, unable to move out of their mental patterns. Instead of allowing thoughts to flow in free association or to progress in an orderly fashion, a person with Spleen difficulties replays the same tapes over and over with very little variation. The problem becomes exacerbated by the fact that, in the Eastern system, both overwork and overthinking damage Spleen function. A vicious circle develops in which rumination decreases Spleen *qi*, which causes more obsessive thought patterns.

Derek had been planning for his upcoming workshop on anxiety for the past three months. He finished his preparation and organization at least two weeks before the talk. However, Derek continued to have obsessive thoughts. He worried about how many people would attend, whether the audiovisual equipment would work, whether the participants would enjoy the food, and whether people would challenge what he had to say about anxiety. Derek found himself checking his notes and the arrangements over and over during the two weeks before the seminar. He even dreamed about there not being enough chairs for people to sit on and their asking ridiculous questions during his presentation.

The *qi* of the Spleen is also responsible for holding things in their place, a metaphorical similarity to the earth's gravitational pull. When Spleen *qi* is at adequate levels, internal organs, blood, and fluids stay where they should. If Spleen *qi* is deficient, the organs prolapse, hemorrhage or bruising results, and urine and semen can leak, in the same manner that objects float once away from the earth's firm control. The holding property of the Spleen can apply to behavior and emotions, as well. Individuals who have problems with staying put or those who can't leave home might have an excess or deficiency of Spleen *qi*. Compulsively putting objects in their place or excessive sloppiness might also reflect Spleen difficulties.

The Stomach is the *yang* organ associated with Earth, and it is connected to the Spleen on many levels. The physiology of the Stomach in the Eastern framework is very close to that of Western medicine, in that it is responsible for receiving and digesting food. The Stomach's ability to function properly is the foundation of health and well-being. If the body ingests positive nutrients and digests them adequately, antipathogenic *qi* is likely to be strong. The *qi* of the Stomach is supposed to flow downward, just as food travels from the mouth to the stomach to the intestine. Disruption of Stomach harmony means that its *qi* becomes "rebellious" and instead moves upward. Belching, regurgitation, and vomiting are all examples of Stomach *qi*'s traveling in the wrong direction.

Each of the five elements relates to a different sense organ, and given its association with eating, it is not surprising that Earth is connected to the mouth and taste. Difficulties with tasting food, chewing, and swallowing are frequently the result of Spleen imbalance.

> Rochelle, a 29-year-old bank teller, presented for therapy. Brian, her husband of 11 years and a childhood sweetheart, had gone off with her best friend. For the past two weeks, Rochelle had been finding it difficult to go to work or even to leave the house. She had very little appetite, and food was generally unappealing. When she did force herself to eat, a strange thing would happen. Rochelle would put the food in her mouth and chew, but she could not bring herself to swallow. Even food that looked appealing had to be held in her mouth for several minutes before she could force herself to move it further. Sometimes she gave up and spit it out in her napkin. Rochelle had lost nine pounds in two weeks, and she was terrified that she might never be able to eat normally again. Therapy was directed toward getting Rochelle to "swallow" what had happened between her husband and her best friend so that she could reinstate healthier eating patterns.

In Eastern healing, Earth "governs the flesh." This means that the element is related to the substantiality of the body. Clients who are overweight or underweight are likely to have an excess or deficiency of Earth energy. This can become manifest as an acute condition, as in the loss of appetite or bingeing following a traumatic event, or as a constitutional weakness. People who have chronic weight problems are likely to have internal Earth imbalances, while those who have a temporary change of body mass are probably responding to external events.

Because of the intrinsic interrelatedness of mind and body, the substantiality of Earth is reflected in thoughts, as well. Clients who have problems with "fleshing" out an idea or who only provide the bare bones of information can have Earth deficiencies. Those who provide "meaty" illustrations with more detail than necessary might be demonstrating an excess of Earth energy.

Helen, a 25-year-old single mother, attended therapy with her four-year-old daughter, Erica. She began by describing how Erica opposed her authority and provided numerous illustrations. The therapist listened thoughtfully for 10 minutes and then suggested some ideas that might be helpful. Helen ignored the input and continued to elucidate details of the problem. She began to repeat the entire history, adding information about how Erica had been disobedient as a baby, crying at night and refusing to be breastfed. Every instance of Erica's misbehavior since that time was recounted, many for a second time. Attempts to stop the recitation were met with irritation, no matter how the therapist tried to validate the severity of Erica's problem.

The fluid related to Earth is saliva, which makes sense given the element's connection to eating and digestion. Excessive drooling can be related to either Spleen excess or deficiency. A deficiency of Spleen *qi* might cause the organ to fail in its role of transportation, resulting in an accumulation of fluids in the mouth. An excess of dampness in the Spleen might produce more fluid than a normal level of *qi* could transport. As is true of any differential diagnosis, other symptoms would have to be considered to distinguish between the two.

Damp is the climatic factor that most disrupts Earth functioning. As in nature, Earth is in its healthiest state when adequate moisture is present. Too much dampness turns the earth muddy and moldy. Spleen energetics are particularly sensitive to high levels of dampness. An excess of cold and damp in the Spleen produces such symptoms as loss of appetite, sticky saliva, diarrhea, fullness and distention in the abdomen, and a white, sticky tongue coating. An excess of damp heat in the Spleen creates the same fullness and distention in the abdomen, but the face and eyes are yellow, the tongue coating is yellow, there are nausea and vomiting, and the body feels heavy.

From a therapy perspective, an excess of damp creates individuals who become stuck and can't move. There is a "heaviness" about their affect, as if their emotions were weighing them down. Issues are often muddied and unclear, and clients have difficulty elucidating them. Action is impossible, not because of a lack of energy, but because the clients seem enveloped in their problems, held in the bog of their dilemma. Even if they want to move, they can't.

> Billie came to therapy despondent and overwhelmed. A 32-year-old attorney, she had recently been hired by a high-powered corporate firm. Billie said that going to work each week to generate 60 billable hours while caring for her two children and trying to maintain a successful marriage was too much. Her desperation was making her depressed, and she felt too swamped to handle anything well. The managing partner of her firm told her that if she wanted to be a successful lawyer, there could be no compromise or letting up. He criticized her for being weak and not pulling her share of the load. Billie's husband, Bo, a successful architect, and her two children said they were worried about her, but also described missing her attention. Her mother criticized her constantly for putting her work before her family. Billie knew she had to do something, but her problems seemed so enormous that she didn't' know where to start. She reviewed the situation mentally, but there didn't seem to be any acceptable solution.

Dampness is probably the most difficult condition to treat because it creates such a high level of immobility. In Eastern healing, treatment centers on removing the cause of the damp, if possible, and then reducing its levels within the system. If the damp is of a cold nature, warmth can be used to dispel it, in the same way that heating a home in the winter can remove dampness and mold. If the damp is of a hot nature, however, adding heat might remove the dampness, but it would cause *yang* levels to become unacceptably high, like turning up a heater on a hot, humid day. An alternative means of dehumidifying needs to be used that will reduce the damp without overheating the problem or chilling the system back into immobility.

From the Eastern perspective, in the healing of damp conditions, treatment modalities are selected that require the least amount of participation by the client. If someone is mired in quicksand, it is of little use asking the person to work his or her way out. The only participation requested of the client is to stop engaging in activities that might be adding to the problem (for example, eating damp foods, such as dairy products or greasy potato chips; using a Jacuzzi; or fly fishing). The balance of the treatment comes from the practitioner. Using acupuncture or herbs, the healer works to move the damp and reduce its levels.

Psychotherapists often struggle with damp clients, trying to get them to act, but with little success. No matter how high their motivation, they can't move sufficiently to follow suggestions or make improvements. Therapy becomes bogged down and improvements are minimal and slow. Both client and therapist become increasingly frustrated by the lack of progress.

A client in this situation is analogous to a car that is stuck in mud. The therapist comes along and encourages the client to rev the engine while the therapist pushes. Sometimes this is sufficient to get things moving, and the client happily moves on. If the mud is extremely deep, however, or the car has been sitting in it for a long time, no amount of pushing or reving is going to free it. While it would be helpful to ask the client to stop doing things that make the car become more enmeshed, he or she might not have sufficient power, even with the therapist's aid, to create action. To fix the situation, the therapist might need to direct the client out through the window or to find other people to help push the car.

Enlisting family members to help "push" can be useful, especially those who aren't mired in the problem or those who might be creating the mud. The therapist can also pursue avenues of redirection, allowing the client to move out of the car and into more productive activities.

Therapy with Billie began by trying to get her to list priorities so that she could start reducing the enormity of her problem. She came back the next week saying that she hadn't found the time to think about the list, much less to complete it. After several other suggestions were discounted as too difficult to pursue, it was agreed that Billie would bring her family to the next session. When they came in for therapy, Bo and the children agreed that making Billie happy was currently their most important consideration. They decided that they would divide among themselves all the responsibilities concerning the home and their own care. Bo would make sure the children were fed and did their homework. The children would clean their own rooms and try to do nice things for their mother when she came home at night. Bo took over paying the bills and became the initiator of all romantic and intimate relations.

After three months of the arrangement, Billie felt that she was functioning at a much better level. She said that she could finally think clearly enough to see that corporate law was not the best career path for her, and she found a position in a small firm that valued her as a person. Over the subsequent months, Billie was able to resume a more participatory role within the family, although she felt comfortable with continuing to delegate some of the responsibility.

Sweet is the flavor associated with Earth. For all of the elements, eating a small amount of food with the associated flavor helps the energy, but overindulging in it creates problems in the element. Individuals who crave sweet foods often have an Earth imbalance, and those who binge on sugary foods often create Spleen difficulties.

In Eastern diagnostics, the odor of a client is also important (one of the four diagnostic categories being listening/smelling). Individuals with Earth imbalances can have a cloyingly sweet smell to their body or discharges (urine, for instance). The sound associated with Earth is singing or humming. Clients with a singsong quality to their voices or who hum constantly might have difficulties with the Earth element.

Contemplation is the emotion associated with Earth. In its healthy form, it exists as an ability to reflect and consider, an almost meditative state. If the element is imbalanced, however, contemplation transforms into rumination. Worrying permeates behavior, and the individual often becomes immobilized by his or her thought patterns. In its most extreme form, rumination develops into compulsions, as thinking narrows to rigid, repetitive patterns. Fixations on certain ideas become evident, and opinions are solidified.

Yellow is the color associated with the element. The skin tone of a client with Earth difficulties can manifest as pale yellow in cold or deficiency problems to bright yellow with heat or excess problems. Some

Eastern practitioners feel that a person's preference for a color is important diagnostically. Those who routinely wear a certain color or who hate a specific hue might have difficulties with the element associated with the color. A client who wears only yellow shirts or one who has recently developed a distaste for yellow foods might have an Earth imbalance. The symptoms should be considered in light of their extremity and relation to other diagnostic information.

Each element is associated with a season of the year. Earth is often linked to late summer, but in many Eastern systems, it is related to seasonal transitions—spring to summer, summer to autumn, etc.—since Earth is the energy of transformation. Problems related to Earth, such as eating difficulties or obsessions, can peak during these changes of season. Similarly, individuals with Earth imbalances can have more difficulty with any type of transition, whether a change in a daily schedule or a shift to daylight saving time.

Dreams can also indicate disharmony in an element. Clients with Spleen imbalances often dream of food, home, or a sense of belongingness. Claustrophobia, a fear of being closed or walled in, or agoraphobia, an inability to leave home, might be indicative of Earth dysfunction.

Depression manifests in different ways, depending on the element that produces it. The imbalance of each element results in a specific distribution of symptoms. Whereas Major Depression is considered a single diagnostic category in Western thought, there are five very different patterns in Eastern healing.

Earth depression is marked by significant changes in eating patterns, either loss of appetite or bingeing. Food is often described as tasteless and unappealing or is used as a source of comfort and nurturance. Acute Spleen depression is marked by changes in weight. In chronic conditions, the individual is routinely heavy or thin. Cravings for or avoidance of sweets is noted. If a suicide attempt occurs, it is often by the ingestion of pills.

High levels of rumination are evident. Clients seem incapable of escaping from their thought patterns into action. They constantly play mental tapes of past interactions or obsess about future events. Their thoughts rarely focus on the present or translate into plans. They become totally self-absorbed and egocentric, living mostly within the confines of their thought patterns.

Individuals with Earth depression find it difficult to form attachments. They aren't able to get out of their heads sufficiently to make a connection or have an interpersonal relationship. Alternatively, they can become obsessively enmeshed with another person, unable to differentiate themselves from the other.

In Earth depression, rituals and cycles become very important. Compulsive patterns emerge, with the person insisting that things and events remain in their proper places. Alternatively, in a deficient pattern, the depressive may show a complete disregard for tidiness, paying no attention to order or schedule.

As discussed previously, if the imbalance has a damp aspect, the depression becomes a chronic pattern, with little or no movement observed. Change is difficult to produce through treatment, and the syndrome seems resistant to therapy. Any improvement is gradual and slight.

The element of Earth has both diagnostic and treatment implications. In subsequent chapters, its relationship to the other four elements, and how this affects intrapersonal and interpersonal therapy, will be considered.

# CHAPTER NINE

## Metal

■

*Oversharpen the blade, and the edge will*
*soon blunt*
*Amass a store of gold and jade, and no*
*one can protect it.*

*—Lao-tzu*

The element of Metal was originally conceptualized as Air. While the two are very different in Western thinking, in the historical Eastern context, both existed as distillations of pure essence. Metal was the crystallization of the essential properties from the earth, while Air was the pure *qi* from heaven. Together they formed the energy that drives all things. Over time, the element came to be called only by the name of Metal, for reasons that will become more apparent in Chapter 13, but the essence of Air remained within the properties of the element.

Metal is both structure and strength, as in the iron and steel that form the foundation or walls of a building. After being extracted from the earth, aspects of a metal can nourish the body (minerals) or adorn it (gold and silver). It gives other substances support and glitter. Metal can be useful or frivolous, but it is always coveted.

The *yin* organ associated with Metal is the Lung. It is in the Lung that *qi* is formed for the entire body. The nutritional essences extracted by the Spleen are sent up to the Lung, where they mix with the pure *qi* breathed in from the air. The process is a metaphor for the creation of metal from the distillations of the earth. The Lung combines the essences, forms them into *qi*, and distributes the *qi* throughout the body. If this dispersal function is impaired by the presence of excess dampness, cold, dryness, or heat, the formation and movement of energy are restricted, and familiar Lung symptoms, such as coughing or wheezing, appear. For there to be healthy, noncontaminated energy in the body, the Lung must perform well. A deficiency of *qi* is often the result of the Lung's lack of success in fulfilling its role.

> Dinah spoke to the therapist in a low voice, barely managing brief responses to any questions, and rarely volunteering information. She seemed vaguely aware of her surroundings, but they didn't interest her greatly. Her breathing was shallow and labored. It appeared that she didn't have the energy even to sit properly in the chair, but leaned on the armrest for support. It was hard to find any topic that created either interest or concern.

In Eastern physiology, the Lung is also responsible for the body's defenses, Metal being both breath and sword. It regulates the defensive *qi* by controlling the opening and closing of the pores of the skin, thus allowing things to enter and leave the body. This protective function prevents the penetration of pathogens (cold, wind, viruses, bacteria, etc.) into the interior of the body. Because it is the first line of defense, the Lung is also the initial organ affected by the invasion of outside influences. Colds and flu are the result of the defensive barrier's being penetrated, and the symptoms associated with them are related to a disruption of Metal's dispersing functions.

Metal also plays a defensive role on an emotional and behavioral level. Individuals who allow anyone and anything into their personal spaces are demonstrating a Lung deficiency. Clients who barricade themselves against any interpersonal involvement often have overprotective defensive energy.

> Victor presented for therapy at the request of his mother, who was worried that her son was not leading a normal life. Victor, 22 years old and working as a dishwasher, didn't understand his mother's concern. He said that his mother always questioned why Victor didn't go out with friends or was never involved with a woman. Victor held himself emotionally separate from his family as well. When asked why he didn't pursue relationships, he

replied that he had watched his mother marry twice and divorce twice. He felt that getting involved with other people was a sure recipe for pain. Victor said that he was fine with spending his time reading and going to work, and that he didn't need or want anything else.

Metal's protective barriers can also be raised against new ideas. Clients who insist on maintaining their views or opinions even in the face of overwhelming evidence to the contrary might have an imbalance in their Metal energetics. Those who won't try anything new or who insist that familiar ways are better might have a dysfunction in this element.

The *yang* organ associated with Metal is the Large Intestine. Its function is elimination, the removal of waste from the body, although the Lung shares some responsibility for removing impurities through the process of exhalation. Problems associated with the accumulation of waste, such as constipation, or abnormalities regarding elimination, such as encopresis, would be associated with the Metal element.

Metal is also involved with discharges of a more emotional and spiritual nature. Individuals who can't let go, whether of feelings or past events, frequently have imbalances in this element. For functioning to be healthy, there must be a normal progression from intake to elimination, retaining essential or desirable components and discharging those that are unnecessary or unwanted. If a person begins to hold on to everything, or to nothing, that is usually a sign that the system is not operating properly. Stubbornness, hoarding, or living in the past are all signs of Metal's not fulfilling its function of elimination.

Candace, a 29-year-old hospital worker, could not get over her ex-boyfriend, Mick. Despite the fact that their relationship had terminated more than two years earlier, she spent all of her time thinking about Mick and reliving their time together. She kept every gift Mick had ever given her, and she spent her free time taking them out and looking at them. Candace refused to consider seeing someone else, and had even terminated friendships when her behavior was questioned. When her sense of loss seemed to overwhelm her, Candace would drive past Mick's house, consoling herself by seeing where he lived or looking at his car. Candace sometimes missed Mick so much that she would skip work to go somewhere that they had visited together.

The sense organ associated with Metal is the nose, a natural extension of its function of respiration. Difficulties with a sense of smell are often indicative of problems in the element. Individuals who are hypersensitive to odors, or who cannot perceive them, often have Lung imbalances.

Metal is also reflected in the skin and body hair. Given its relation to defense, it makes sense that the Lung is connected to the external barriers of the body. Metal often protects the body by opening and closing the pores of the skin, and shutting out pathogens when necessary. If unwanted toxins need to be eliminated, they can be released through sweat, the fluid associated with Metal. Clients who perspire abundantly often have deficient Lung *qi*, the energy being insufficient to hold the fluid in its place or to close the pores properly. People who are thin-skinned (overly sensitive to problems) or are thick-skinned (resistant to influence) exhibit metaphorical aspects of the function of Metal.

Skin diseases can also indicate a problem with the Metal element. Such problems sometimes develop because impurities are not being properly eliminated through the bowel or lungs and instead emerge from the skin. At other times, the skin reflects conditions of imbalance, such as excess damp or heat in the interior of the body.

Dryness is the climatic factor related to Metal. Steel is most flexible in a molten state; it becomes rigid and brittle when it dries out. For the Lung and Large Intestine to function well, sufficient, but not excess, moisture should be present. An overabundance of dryness disrupts both Metal organs—the Lung becomes unable to moisten the skin properly or distribute *qi*, and the Large Intestine is not able to lubricate stools enough for them to pass.

Smoking cigarettes dries out the lungs and destroys their *yin* aspect. Smokers often report a "buzz" from a cigarette, followed by a later craving. This occurs because smoking creates a false-heat situation (normal levels of *yang* but deficient levels of *yin*). The disproportionate amount of heat feels like a burst of energy, as the cooling, stabilizing factors decrease. The relatively higher levels of heat can also stimulate digestive activity and decrease damp, leading to a reduction of weight, even with an increase in appetite. Unfortunately, the *yang* symptoms produced by smoking are a false rather than a true effect. The positive feelings are a mirage that must be repeated endlessly to maintain the illusion. More significantly, the lack of balancing *yin* creates difficulties within the Lung, leading to such internal diseases as cancer and emphysema.

From a therapy perspective, dryness often presents as brittleness. It is as if a person's nourishing, moistening aspects have evaporated, leaving that person fragile and crackly. Emotionally, the individual has dried up, ready to shatter at the slightest touch. Metaphorically, he or she is like a sheet of metal, rusted and dry. The least pressure can cause the once substantial structure to flake into a multitude of pieces.

Zena attended therapy at the request of the Child Protection Agency because of concerns that she was neglecting her two children, Dan, age eight and Bruce, age six. Although only 25, Zena looked much older. Her husband, Stu, had left her two years earlier. Zena didn't miss Stu's violent behavior, but she was worried that he would kidnap her children with the support of her own parents, who had sided with him during the divorce proceedings.

Zena appeared nervous and shaky during the first session. She was generally unresponsive to the therapist and looked as though she would break down if pressed to answer questions. She kept her body hunched forward, almost as if protecting herself from the therapist. After much patient prodding, Zena described her life as a runaway adolescent when she worked as a prostitute to support herself. Her husband had taken her off the streets and into a more normal environment, which was why she stayed with Stu even when he was abusive. Zena was very wary during the session, seeing the therapist as an extension of the Child Protection Agency, despite assurances to the contrary.

Dryness is best treated by adding moisture, or *yin*. In a therapy context, this usually entails finding something that moistens and nourishes, an intervention that makes the person more fluid and adaptable. It is important that, in cases of extreme dryness, the treatment doesn't rush in as a torrent, shattering the brittle structure or failing to penetrate its exterior. The desert floor cannot accept the rain from a sudden storm; the water rolls off its surface and causes flooding. Moisture is best introduced slowly enough to be absorbed.

Several sessions later, Zena's twin sister was brought into therapy, after Zena had commented that Zoe was the one person she didn't find threatening.

Zena hadn't seen her sister since leaving home years earlier, but she had fond memories of her. Session time was spent allowing the sisters to connect and reestablish their relationship. Gradually, Zena began to relax during therapy and become more open. With her sister's help, she engaged in some play with her children and discussed ways in which she could parent them better.

The flavors associated with Metal are pungent and spicy. Again, eating a small amount of the flavor can strengthen the functioning of the element, but overindulgence in hot foods, such as chilies, curry, or pepper, will cause problems. A client who craves or avoids spicy food usually has a Metal imbalance. The odor associated with Metal is "rotten," and individuals with severe difficulties with the element give off that particular smell. The sound connected with the element is whining. Clients who nasalize their speech or who whine their complaints frequently have Metal types of problems.

White is the color associated with the element. This can be reflected in pallor of the skin or the color of the tongue coating. If a client either dresses only in white or detests the color, that could be a sign of Metal imbalance. Autumn is the season associated with the element. Many colds, flus, and skin problems appear at this time, and clients with the emotional or energy difficulties related to Metal may find their symptoms exacerbated during this season.

The emotion most significantly linked to the Metal element is grief, since one of the things a Metal personality can hold onto inappropriately is sadness. Imbalances in this element often create an inability to pass out of the grieving process. In an ideal world, clients who experience loss should be able eventually to let go of their grief and resume healthy functioning. Individuals with problems in the Metal aspect grieve endlessly or inappropriately. The depths of their melancholy are extreme and can be triggered by insignificant events.

Lisa, age 74, had lost her husband, Russell, to cancer eight years previously. Shortly after his death, Lisa retired from teaching, sold her house, and moved to a home for seniors. She rarely interacts with the other residents, preferring to spend her days and nights alone, surrounded by pictures of herself and Russell during their time together. Efforts by the staff to involve her in other activities are usually ignored. Lisa is in generally good health, with the exception of a susceptibility to colds and chronic constipation. Her children and grandchildren visit her frequently, and although she enjoys their company, she tires quickly and lacks the energy to communicate for very long. Her children worry about her despondency, but any efforts to get Lisa motivated have proved unsuccessful.

Grieving problems are exacerbated by Metal's relationship to *qi*. Clients who have deficiencies in that element often do not have the energy to pull themselves out of their despair. Therapy that uses interventions that require action or movement is unsuccessful because the client does not have sufficient *qi* to comply. As discussed previously, in deficient-*qi* situations, energy often needs to be added before the client can act.

Dreams involving the color white indicate Metal disharmony, as do those of flying and cruel killings. Phobias about air and breathing, such as a fear of flying or suffocation, could be related to Metal. Acts of self-mutilation involving cutting can be indicative of a Metal imbalance, particularly if they are emotionally linked to grief or sadness, or to a difficulty with holding onto things or people.

Carrie, age 14, had lost her mother the previous year in an automobile accident. She and her 12-year-old sister were forced to move in with their estranged father, a man with whom they had not had contact since they were young children. Carrie felt that her father was not capable of understanding her since he barely knew her. She presented for therapy after she began to make scratches on her forearm with a knife. Carrie says that she cuts herself out of frustration. She misses her mother's understanding and coping skills. Carrie prays every night for her mother's return, and then ritualistically marks herself.

The Metal form of depression is marked by energy depletion and high levels of fatigue. The client is often unwilling or unable to speak, not having the *qi* to express his or her feelings, and if the client does talk, the voice is low or whiny. Breathing is often shallow or ragged. There is frequently a sense of loss or grief. Such clients feel isolated, sensing or placing a barrier between themselves and other people. At times, this manifests as the idea that they differ from everyone around them, that no one feels or thinks the same as they do. They may mark or pierce their skin in symbolic fashion, in the form either of tattoos or self-harm. If they commit suicide, it is often by hanging or suffocation.

The contrast between Earth and Metal depression is dramatic. Rumination and eating difficulties mark the former, whereas lack of energy and melancholy distinguish the latter. Depression emerges as a multidimensional concept requiring differentiation for both diagnosis and treatment. Cognitive-behavior therapies, for example, should work considerably better with an Earth depression, where there is a high level of rumination, than with a Metal depression. For treatment to be effective, a differential diagnosis of the problem is essential.

# CHAPTER TEN

## Water

■

*The highest good is like water.*
*Water gives life to the ten thousand things*
*and does not strive.*
*It flows in places men reject and so is like*
*the Tao.*

—*Lao-tzu*

Water is quintessential *yin* energy. It is the primary component of life on the earth—sustaining, refreshing, maintaining. Water has substance, but it constantly changes in relation to its surroundings. The form of water is the shape of the container. But water is not always a passive guest. It sculpts the structures that hold it, as in the formation of a canyon or the erosion of a shore. It can adapt to the environment or mold it.

The energy of water is a spectrum, from stagnant pool to pounding ocean. It can be both a bubbling spring and a vast lake, a drop from a canteen or a raging rapid. Too little water means death, but an excess can drown you. Water is freshest when flowing and becomes rank when stagnant.

The Kidney and Bladder are the organs related to Water. Like most *yang* organs, the Bladder is the less significant of the pair; its function is very similar to that in Western physiology, to store urine and release it when needed. Problems with difficult urination or enuresis can be related to Bladder functioning. A careful differential diagnosis has to be made because the Spleen is also related to the transportation of fluids. If other Earth signs are present, such as eating difficulties or digestive problems, the urinary problems might be due to deficient Spleen energy rather than to problems with the Bladder.

The *yin* organ associated with Water, the Kidney, is one of the most important organs and the root of Eastern physiology. The function and well-being of the Kidney affect all of the other organs of the body and the core health of the individual—in part, because it is the place where *jing*, the essential essence, is stored. Remember that *jing* is both inherited and acquired. The congenital core is enveloped by a protective coating of acquired *jing* generated by healthy living. If stress or a fast-lane lifestyle consumes the acquired essence, the inherited *jing* becomes exposed and vulnerable. The Kidney is the treasure house of the body, holding and guarding vital resources. If the sentry is asleep or slow, the jewels of the kingdom can disappear.

*Jing* is the *yin* facet of the Kidney. Its *yang* component is known as *ming men*, life gate fire. It might seem paradoxical for Water to have a fiery aspect, but within the deepest recesses of *yin*, one finds a core of *yang*, the contrasting dot of white in the black half of the *taiqitu* symbol. *Ming men* is the pilot light of the body; its heat is the source of all energy and function. The life gate fire also drives proper growth and development. In the Eastern system, dwarfism, developmental delays, and premature aging are all related to this aspect of Kidney function.

The health of the Kidney can be monitored through the teeth, bones, and head hair. *Jing* creates marrow, the inner core of bone, so the growth and strength of bones are related to Kidney energy. An individual with stunted growth or easily shattered bones might have a Water imbalance. The shrinkage and hunching of old age are a product of declining Kidney *qi*. Teeth are considered the excess of bone, and their health depends on adequate levels of *jing*.

The brain is also related to the Kidney via the marrow. The ability to think clearly and well is an indication that Water is healthy. The dementia associated with old age is a product of declining Kidney strength. Head hair is the "sprout" of the Kidney. If *jing* is being maintained at healthy levels, the hair is full, shiny, and black (remember, this is an Oriental system; black can be reframed as "dense in color"). If the Kidney's energetics are failing or *jing* is consumed, the hair becomes sparse, falls out, or turns white.

Hannah came for treatment with her 10-month-old son, Sean. Sean had suffered digestive difficulties since birth, with each feeding followed by severe diarrhea or vomiting. His doctor felt that Sean suffered from a wide range of food allergies, which prevented him from ingesting either formula or food directly. Even when breastfed, Sean reacted to the foods that Hannah ate. His symptoms became so serious and his weight loss so extreme that Hannah was restricted to eating only chicken, rice, and bananas, as these produced the least negative consequences for her son. At the time of treatment, Hannah weighed only 92 pounds, and so was very emaciated for her height of five feet, nine inches. Her skin was sallow and there were dark circles under her eyes. Over the past six months, her hair had begun to gray dramatically. Hannah's teeth had also become so loose that they moved in her gums. She complained of an inability to think clearly and only made it through her day by adhering to a familiar schedule.

In Hannah's case, restricted eating had caused a severe depletion of core essence and energy. Her *jing* had already been reduced by Sean's delivery (women lose *jing* through childbirth), and her restricted food intake while trying to nurse her son had led to a further consumption of her core resources.

The Kidney opens to the ear and the "anterior and posterior orifices" (the genitals and anus). The loss of hearing with age is a reflection of declining Kidney function. Tinnitus, particularly the type of ringing or buzzing that stops when a finger is placed in the ear, is often a sign of deficient Kidney *qi*. On a behavioral level, an inability to listen to another or to hear what the person has to say can indicate an imbalance in the Water element.

The Mullins family attended therapy for help with communication issues. Both of the sons—Jake, 14, and Larry, 12—felt that their father, Sam, did not care about them as he never heard anything they said. They stated that their father's typical response to them was "Huh?," which only caused them to repeat information that he would not listen to yet again. Their mother, Janet, defended her husband, saying that he was under stress at work and preoccupied with selling enough insurance to support his family. Sam Mullins was in a daze for most of the session, often asking his wife to repeat for him what had happened. He said that his hearing was fine, but that his work tired him, and what energy he had left, he used to mentally plan his appointments for the next day.

The function of the genitals, whether for urination or sexuality, is also integrally related to Kidney energetics. A deficiency of Kidney *qi* means that there is insufficient energy to hold things in their place and can cause dribbling urine, incontinence, a leakage of sperm, or premature ejaculation. Impotence and infertility are also related to Kidney *qi* and *jing* since adequate levels of both are required for producing an erection or conception. If the Kidney has a deficiency of *yin*, its moistening component, vaginal dryness or insufficient ejaculation can result.

Trudy, a 42-year-old executive, presented for therapy with Max, her husband of 15 years. They were having problems in their relationship because Trudy no longer had much interest in sex. Max said that in the earlier stages of their marriage, they had maintained an adequate level of intimacy, but in recent years, the sex had just stopped. Trudy said that she still loved her husband dearly, and there was no one else. Even when she traveled alone to acquire art for her museum projects, she was not tempted to have an affair. Trudy knew her husband had desires, but she didn't feel that she had the interest or energy to satisfy him.

In Eastern medicine, the Kidney also has the role of grasping *qi* and pulling it down to the lower parts of the body. While the Lung produces *qi* and disperses it, the Kidney assists the process by carrying the energy to the root of the body. The difference in the roles of the two organs can best be seen in relation to asthma. In a "Kidney" type of asthma, the individual has problems with inhalation; he or she can't breathe deeply enough because the organ is not fulfilling its function of pulling the *qi* down. In "Lung" asthma, breathing in is fine, but the person has problems with exhalation, feeling unable to push sufficient air out of the lungs or to do so smoothly. As Kidney asthma is usually the result of deficient *qi*, exercise or exertion makes the problem worse; the increased expenditure of energy creates a further deficit of *qi*. Lung asthma is often an excess condition that results when too much damp or dryness prevents the organ from actualizing its function of expelling waste and air.

If the Lung is generating a sufficient level of energy, but the Kidney cannot grasp it, the *qi* cannot reach the interior core of the individual. A client with this pattern often feels driven, but upon starting to work or exercise, he or she quickly becomes exhausted. The chest feels full and constricted as energy accumulates, but the lower back and knees are achy and tired. The client often interprets these as symptoms of generalized anxiety, restlessness, or chronic fatigue.

According to *The Yellow Emperor's Inner Classic*, written about 100 B.C., the developmental pattern generated by the Kidney follows a seven-year cycle in women and an eight-year cycle in men. Water energy first flowers in girls at the age of seven and at eight in boys, creating a burst of hair growth and the emergence of permanent teeth. At 14 and 16, puberty flourishes, resulting in fertility and sexuality. At 21 and 24, respectively, the Kidney is fully active, with the emergence of the wisdom teeth marking the process, and sexual energies robust. At 28 and 32, the *qi* of the Kidney peaks, and the bones finish their growth. The decline of Kidney energetics begins at 35 for women and at 40 for men, with the face starting to wrinkle and the hair thinning out. By 42 and 48, the face is lined even more and the hair whitens. At 49 and 56, reproductive energy diminishes, particularly in women; the muscles begin to slacken and hearing declines. *The Yellow Emperor's Inner Classic* ceases its age associations at this point, a product of either the likelihood of a short life span or the horror of life without an adequate supply of *jing*. As has been documented since, as the decline in Kidney energy continues, the body dries up, the bones shrink, and vital essence disappears. The decline is faster if stress or an unhealthy lifestyle has consumed *jing* at a higher rate. For the pattern to be delayed, *jing* and *qi* must be cultivated and protected through beneficial and restorative living.

The emotion related to Water is fear. An excess of the element can make one rigid with apprehension; a deficiency might create fainting or urinary incontinence. Generalized anxiety or apprehension might be an indication that the cooling, nurturing aspect of Water is inadequate.

Terry, age nine, and his family came to therapy for help with his fears and enuresis. Terry was afraid of walking up or down stairs, of catching a ball, and of talking to other children at school. His behavior was in stark contrast to that of his younger brothers, Andrew and Charles, who were socially active and fearless. Terry's father indicated that he himself had been timid as a child, although Terry's mother had never been phobic. The parents said Terry's fears had been present since early childhood, but lately were becoming worse. Terry wet his bed every night, and if he felt pressured at school, would have urinary accidents there as well.

Ambition and will are the positive aspects of Water energetics. Clients who seem driven or unshakable are Water personalities. In a healthy state, this manifests as the energy and ability to pursue work, interests, or goals. When there is an imbalance in Water, however, the client's drive seems more like a flood, sweeping away or destroying anything in its path.

Cassandra, a wife and the mother of three children, presented for therapy, deeply unhappy in her marriage. She said that her husband, Charles, had refused to attend with her, considering the sessions a waste of time and money. Charles was feared by both his family and coworkers. He had established his first business at the age of 19, and by 32, was the head of a network of delivery companies. He had made his first million dollars by underselling one of his cousins, forcing the older man out of business and into bankruptcy. When his mother pleaded with him to show some compassion, Charles had laughingly asked her how to spell the word. He rarely saw his wife or children, and when he was home, everyone was expected to coddle him or to disappear. Cassandra had endured his behavior for the sake of her security and children. Recently, however, Charles had become annoyed when Cassandra sent her parents an anniversary present, saying that their money was not to be squandered on frivolous items. He took her checkbook and refused to let her have any money other than what he gave her each day. The only reason Charles had agreed to allocate funds for therapy was that Cassandra had threatened an expensive divorce.

Cold is the climatic factor that most adversely affects Water, freezing it and impeding motion. In cold weather, sweating decreases, and the kidneys must work harder to process fluids as urine. Cold exacerbates problems with the life gate fire, so sexual problems become worse and energy decreases when the client is chilled. In extreme cases, this presents as frigidity or being "frozen" with fear. It makes sense that winter is the season related to Water, and bones ache more with the cold.

Prevention is the best way to avoid Water difficulties, since *jing* cannot be replaced once lost. A healthy lifestyle and moderate sexual practices conserve and protect essential energy. No amount of treatment can restore *jing*. If the essential essence is not harmed, however, Kidney energy can be replenished by providing warmth, rest, and nourishment.

Terry, the fearful nine-year-old enuretic, spoke to the therapist in a low voice, expressing a desire to get rid of some of his fears and to stop having accidents. A program was set in place whereby he would be gradually exposed to his fears without any pressure to resolve them. His father took him to the local mall, and walked up and down the stairs with his son whenever Terry felt he wanted to try. After each attempt, he would buy his son a small present or sit with him watching the people. At school, the counselor and teacher arranged for several of the more popular boys to spend time with Terry, including sitting with him at lunch. One of the boys even offered to teach Terry how to catch a ball, telling him that he had had trouble until his father showed him a neat trick. Gradually, Terry felt more comfortable at school, and the urinary accidents stopped, although he continued to wet his bed occasionally at night.

The sound associated with Water is groaning, and clients with imbalances often moan about their problems. The color related to the element is black. Clients with Kidney difficulties often have dark circles under their eyes or hollows in their cheeks. Dreams of water or ships can be related to the element.

Salty is the flavor associated with Water. Once again, eating a small amount of the related substance strengthens the element. An overconsumption of salt disrupts the Kidney's ability to process fluids, and such problems as edema or high blood pressure can result. The smell related to Water is putrid, as in dead fish being left to rot in a pail of water. Individuals with Kidney failure often have such an odor coming from their bodies.

Water depression is marked by a lack of will and a high level of fear.

There is a diminution of sexual interest and/or sexual dysfunction. The client's demeanor is generally cold and withdrawn. The face is pallid, with dark circles under the eyes. Because of their lack of will, such persons are easily led, although they often don't have the energy to follow through on therapeutic suggestions or interventions. Suicide attempts may involve giving up the will to live or drowning.

# CHAPTER ELEVEN

## Wood

■

*A man is born gentle and weak.*
*At his death he is hard and stiff.*
*Green plants are tender and filled with sap.*
*At their death they are withered and dry.*
*Therefore the stiff and unbending is the disciple of death.*
*The gentle and yielding is the disciple of life*

*.—Lao-tzu*

Trees live with their feet on the ground and their heads in the clouds. They are both rooted and reaching, fixed and mobile. Their bark protects the inner core from unwanted intruders; their leaves are open doorways to the outside. Like humans, they live on the earth, but reach for the heavens.

The ideal essence of Wood in Eastern medicine is that of the young forest—trees that are strong enough to withstand predators, but sufficiently flexible to bend rather than break in strong winds. Trees, like humans, are at their best when they can hold their ground, but still adjust to prevailing influences.

Wood is considered the energy of growth, of "coming out," of free movement. It is responsible for the free flow of energy, the patency of *qi*, throughout the body. When *qi* moves easily, a person feels energetic and well, with an even temperament and the flexibility to adapt to varying situations.

The two main organs in the Eastern medical system that are related to Wood are the Liver and the Gall Bladder. Together they work to ensure that *qi* flows smoothly through the body. On a spiritual level, the Liver is in charge of planning, so difficulties in organization or foresight are attributed to imbalances in that organ. The Gall Bladder assists with decision making, so an inability to select alternatives or a dogged determination to follow only one course of action is suggestive of problems there.

Neil presented for therapy as a 24-year-old graduate student about to finish his studies. He felt totally overwhelmed by the decisions facing him. He had been seeing Ann for the past three years, and she wanted to get married when they finished school. Neil said he loved Ann, but he didn't know whether he wanted the restriction of marriage at this time. He also couldn't visualize life without her. Neil was concerned about his career path as well. He had received job offers from two private-sector firms and one government agency. The more Neil listed the pros and cons of each choice, the more confused he became.

The energy of Wood manifests in the eyes. The difficulties related to eye problems, such as conjunctivitis or cataracts, are indicative of imbalance in the element, but so, too, are problems of vision in a more philosophical sense, as in someone who can't see the forest for the trees. Wood is also related to the tendons and muscles. Like the young trees of the forest, the body is at its best when the limbs are flexible and well nourished. Spasms and poor muscle tone are related to poor Wood functioning, as are problems with emotional inflexibility or stiffness.

Tears are the fluid related to Wood, in part because of its association with the eyes. Inappropriate crying (too much or too little) is often a sign of Wood imbalance. As would be expected, green is the color related to the element, with skin casts and clothing choices indicative of constitutional or current problems.

Wind is the climatic factor, so that individuals with Wood imbalances usually experience an exacerbation of difficulties on windy days. Alternatively, problems that act like the wind, shifting from one place to the other, gusting and dying down, can be related to Wood. A client who moves issues constantly, pains that come and go, or symptoms that flare up and then disappear could all be construed as wind-related problems.

Elaine came for supervision because she was having problems with some difficult cases. She began with a client who was anorexic, but halfway through her report, she diverted her attention to a case involving a schizophrenic who had returned to live with his family. This presentation rapidly evolved into a discussion of an older male client who refused to acknowledge that Elaine had any status as a clinician. The supervisor was unable to keep any of the cases straight, and questioned whether Elaine could. She dissolved into tears, apologizing for her distraction. Her marriage had broken up a few weeks earlier, and Elaine said that she hadn't really been herself since then. The supervisor suggested that while she was feeling stressed, Elaine would be better off concentrating on one small thing at a time. He returned to the case of the anorexic and helped Elaine focus on developing a strategy for that client.

Wood is related to rancid smells and sour tastes. An individual who craves or avoids lemons, vinegar, or sauerkraut could be having an imbalance of the element. The health of the organs associated with Wood, the Liver and Gall Bladder, manifests in the nails. Individuals whose toenails have green tinges (remember, green is also indicative of Wood) or whose fingernails split easily are probably having difficulty with the element. Dreams related to wood and forests, as well as to the color green, are obviously connected to Wood, but the acupuncture classics also include dreams of exhaustion and mushrooms as being relevant.

The emotional components associated with Wood are produced by the element's relationship to the free flow of *qi* in the body. Anger is the primary emotion related to Wood, and shouting is the relevant tone of voice. When the smooth movement of energy is obstructed, tension and heat build, in the same manner that a dam generates power by blocking a river. Since the normal flow of Wood is upward, like that of a tree, and the natural tendency is for heat to rise, the pent-up energy ascends to explode as temper, complete with red eyes, shouting, and a pounding in the head. Other physical symptoms might include vertigo, migraine, tinnitus that becomes worse when the fingers are placed in the ears, and a rapid pulse.

Anthony was feared by his family and the community. A 35-year-old part-time truck driver and part-time gang member, he intimidated his wife by periodically beating her, his two teenage daughters, and his 10-year-old son. One of the daughters, Briana, required hospitalization for psychiatric problems. Anthony had been arrested for attempted murder, but the case was dropped when the witnesses disappeared. He justified his behavior by blaming it on alcohol. Anthony said that drinking makes him go crazy. He feels his head start to pound, and it won't stop until he lashes out at someone. Anthony asked the therapist to teach his family to respect him and his moods. He said that his father had beaten him whenever he misbehaved, and that his mother had also had a drinking problem. Anthony felt that if he could show respect for his parents, his children should do the same for him.

A number of external factors can cause the obstruction of Wood *qi*, most notably, eating too much greasy food or the excessive use of alcohol or cigarettes. Fried food, because it is not easily digestible, tends to clog the system and keep *qi* from circulating. In Eastern, as in Western, medicine, the Liver is responsible for storing and detoxifying the blood. Because of this, alcohol is particularly deleterious to smooth Wood functioning, and, since the nature of alcohol is also "hot," its intake tends to produce anger.

The same parallels are true on an emotional/behavioral level. Frustration can obstruct the flow of *qi* and result in acting out or anger. Similarly, interactive patterns that suppress rather than allow for good communication often erupt into violent, emotional exchanges when tension builds to a sufficient level.

Tim, age 35, and Sharon, age 33, came to marital therapy complaining of serious difficulties in their relationship. They both had well-paying, stimulating jobs, Tim as an architect in a prestigious firm and Sharon as a clinical psychologist in private practice. They enjoyed a good social life with their many friends. The couple's only problem seemed to be that their arguments had become violent lately, with screaming and even physical confrontations. This upset their two daughters, seven-year-old Terry and five-year-old Samantha, who often had to try to separate their parents to keep them from hurting each other.

Tim professed to be confused about the whole situation. He said that he and Sharon usually got along fine, with no arguments or squabbles. However, one moment, everything would be quiet, but the next thing he knew, Sharon would become hysterical and throw things at him. Tim would respond in kind, and they would end up in a fight. As soon as the argument was over, their lives became normal once again. Sharon sat sulkily during Tim's description. When questioned by the therapist, she said that her picture of their marriage wasn't nearly so rosy. Tim did a number of very annoying things, including making her feel bad that her late working hours kept her from putting the kids to bed. Sharon felt that the efforts she made to adjust her schedule, including always being there to send the girls off to school, weren't appreciated by Tim.

The therapist asked Sharon how she normally communicated her dissatisfaction to Tim. She replied that Tim never did much talking, preferring peace and quiet to confrontation, so she didn't like to annoy him with small matters. She kept her feelings to herself, or else left the room to read a book. Sharon commented that Tim never responded to her departure, or even questioned why she was no longer there. Tim countered that he assumed that Sharon was perfectly capable of deciding where she wanted to be and when she wanted to be there. He added that Sharon also did things that annoyed him, but he didn't see the point in arguing constantly, especially when their fighting seemed to be so violent.

The therapist suggested that things might not become so heated if the issues were dealt with in smaller, discrete units. The couple was asked to specify one thing that each would want the other to do for him or her. Tim stated that he would like Sharon to take 10 minutes when she first came home and listen to how his day had gone. Sharon said that she would appreciate a short neck-and-back massage so that she could unwind from her day. They each agreed to meet the other's request. The therapist also suggested that Tim and Sharon choose a song, one that they both liked, which expressed a longing and need for love. They laughed and said they knew of a Willie Nelson tune that fit the bill perfectly. Since neither wanted to confront the other verbally over small issues, whenever they felt deprived or annoyed, they were to play the song over and over, until the other person noticed and responded with an affectionate gesture.

At the next session, Sharon and Tim reported no more violent episodes, although the Willie Nelson song had been played more times than they could stand. The couple felt their problems were resolved, and therapy was terminated.

The couple's violent outbursts were the product of repeatedly suppressing communication so that their resulting frustration blocked the flow of energy in the relationship. An upsurge of heat and anger can also be a "false heat" situation, one caused by normal levels of *yang*, but insufficient cooling *yin* energy. In these cases, the individual is not usually as aggressive or intensely angry as in the true liver fire situation, and there is also an inherent fragility or weakness. The situation is diagnostically similar to what women experience during menopause, with a "hot flash" and agitation, followed by a sudden cooling and tiredness. The heat feels real, but it passes quickly, and the underlying deficiency is exposed.

The difference between true- and false-heat Liver conditions can be seen behaviorally in ADHD children. Individuals with the excess liver-fire type of ADHD are often hyperkinetic, prone to violent temper outbursts in which their faces turn bright red, and have difficulty settling down. Children with false-heat ADHD often seem pale and frail, and experience enuresis or poor memory. Their movements are often agitated, rather than hyperkinetic. Both of these Wood types of ADHD are in contrast to the Fire form of ADHD marked by mental agitation, insomnia, and manic motor patterns.

If the movement of energy is not completely obstructed, but there is enough blockage to keep the *qi* from flowing smoothly, one experiences irritability rather than actual anger. The stagnation of Liver *qi* produced in this situation is frequently an underlying cause of such conditions as premenstrual syndrome and depression. Symptoms of the former, such as breast distention and uneven moods, are produced by the Liver's not being able to fulfill its function of moving the *qi* smoothly, allowing it to collect in some locations (the breasts and intercostal rib area are related to the Liver channel in acupuncture) or flow erratically.

The Wood form of depression is marked by qualities related to the element. The individual often feels frustrated and irritable, with a constant sense that there are obstacles in his or her path of action, a metaphorical manifestation of the blockages of *qi* within. Wood depressives often have vision problems in both a real and an abstract sense, as they complain of blurry sight, and also usually cannot see a way out of their problems. They cry frequently and are generally inflexible in their behavior. Because of the role of the Liver and Gall Bladder in planning and decision making, Wood depressives either are incapable of formulating solutions or vacillate among several courses of action. Suicide attempts are usually dramatic expressions of frustration or anger.

Tony, a 25-year-old actor, was referred to therapy by his family doctor because of his growing depression. Although Tony was successful in local theatre, he was finding it difficult to break into the national scene, having been rejected at his last four auditions for important roles. Tony supported himself on some residual royalties he received from commercials and by working as a waiter. In recent weeks, however, he was so depressed over his failed auditions that he often didn't show up for his job.

Tony's father, a retired actor, now taught drama at a local institution. Tony's mother was supportive of his desire to act, but his father was critical of his decision to follow in the father's footsteps, as he didn't think that his son had the fortitude to sustain him through the ups and downs of an acting career. Tony himself was ambivalent about whether he should continue acting, and he would often schedule auditions and then not show up. He had also begun calling in sick at his job and was in danger of losing it. His girlfriend of two years had left him because, she said, she was tired of his moodiness and irritability. She had also complained that Tony was unable to commit to anything, whether it was where to go to dinner or if they should move in together. Tony expressed frustration because his life was falling apart around him, but there didn't seem to be anything he could do about it.

In cases of Wood-type depression, it is important to decrease the frustrations that are causing the stagnation of *qi*. By reinstating the flow of energy, the client is able to feel less irritable and more goal oriented.

The therapist arranged with Tony to bring his parents to the next session. Tony alternated between snapping at them when they made a comment and crying when they tried to be supportive. The family finally agreed to a plan that would have the parents act as helpers to get Tony functioning again. Tony would move back into the family home temporarily. His mother would wake him up each morning, feed him a nourishing breakfast, and help him plan his day. His father would discuss acting with him every afternoon when he got home from work. Every evening, his brother would drive him to the restaurant where he waited tables.

After several more sessions with the family, Tony reported that he was getting out of bed more easily and that he enjoyed his conversations about acting with his father. He said that he had lost his job as a waiter, but his brother had helped him to find another one. His brother had also accompanied him to an acting class, and was impressed by how respectfully Tony had been treated. The praise he received in class convinced Tony to audition for a regional theater production, and he won the part he wanted. A few weeks into rehearsal, Tony felt that he might try to move back into his own apartment, as he would be getting support from his acting colleagues.

# CHAPTER TWELVE

## Fire

■

*The space between heaven and earth is*
*like a bellows.*
*The shape changes but not the form;*
*The more it moves, the more it yields*
*—Lao-tzu*

Fire is the quintessential *yang* energy. It is movement, warmth, and light. Fire provides the spark to life. Without fire, there is no vitality or passion, no love or compassion. Fire lacks substance but it has a substantial presence. The production of fire requires the consumption of another material; its warmth requires a sacrifice. Fire is the catalyst between matter and energy.

There are four organs related to Fire in the Eastern system. Two of them are *yang* organs, the Small Intestine and the Triple Heater. The Triple Heater has no anatomical structure; its essence is pure function. It regulates the balance of temperature and warmth throughout the body, serving as a thermostatic control. The Triple Heater divides the trunk of the body into three sections: the Upper Heater covers the chest; the Middle Heater, the abdomen, down to the navel; and the Lower Heater, the area below the umbilicus. The Triple Heater serves as a regulator and passageway for water and *qi* through the body, and its physiology is related to the organs located in each section—Heart and Lung in the Upper Heater, Stomach and Spleen in the Middle Heater, and Bladder and Intestines in the Lower Heater. Not many aspects of the Triple Heater apply to therapy, although people who segment or compartmentalize their lives, who don't make transitions easily, or who don't have a sense of balance and well-being might have difficulties in that organ.

The other *yang* organ associated with Fire is the Small Intestine. This organ receives food from the stomach and continues the digestive process by further separating the pure, nutritional essences from the residues. The Small Intestine absorbs the beneficial materials and sends the waste to the Bladder and Large Intestine for excretion. This extraction process is important in a physical sense, but it is vital on an emotional and spiritual level. A healthy Small Intestine allows an individual to perceive relevance and value. Those who cannot discriminate the "pure" from the "impure," and so are susceptible to every fad and fashion, generally have a deficiency in the Small Intestine.

Celeste called herself an eclectic therapist. She read all of the journals related to her field, and even some from other areas to provide a different slant. Celeste prided herself on the number of continuing-education credits she acquired each year as she would attend every seminar that came to town. The back of her business card read like a directory of therapeutic styles, from TA to REBT, CBT to TFT, and it was difficult to tell whether she was practicing therapy or generating random letter combinations. Her favorite therapy was the one covered by the most recent talk she attended. Celeste flitted from supervisor to supervisor, always sure that someone new would give her the insight she sought.

The two *yin* organs related to Fire are the Heart and the Pericardium. The pericardium is the membrane that covers the heart, and its function in Eastern medicine is to protect the heart from harm. Individuals who are wounded easily, in the sense of frequently having their feelings hurt, might have problems with the Pericardium.

The Heart is by far the most significant of all the Fire organs, equaling the Kidney in its importance to the body. As the ultimate essence of *yin* and *yang*, the Kidney and Heart form the root of all health and function. As in Western physiology, the Heart is responsible for moving blood throughout the body. The continuous supply of *xue* allows the tissues and organs to be nourished, creating a rosy complexion and good vitality. All bodily functions depend on the uninterrupted flow of blood. If the process is disrupted for any reason, as in a stroke, a cardiac block, or hemorrhage, the area not receiving *xue* fails to be nourished and can die or atrophy.

For psychotherapists, the Heart's most significant function is that of "housing" the mind and *shen*. The Heart governs all mental activities, and so thinking, memory, and consciousness are all related to the organ. Individuals who exhibit disrupted thought patterns, hallucinations, poor memory, or dissociation are likely to be having problems with Fire.

> Bruce and his wife, Jill, came to therapy. Jill said Bruce was making her crazy by asserting that she was having an affair with his best friend, Moe. Bruce would badger her for information, telling her that he had evidence from a number of local hotels attesting to the fact that she and Moe had stayed there. He would never supply details, but he swore that he could provide statements from several desk clerks. Even when Jill furnished concrete evidence that she had been with a friend or at home with their daughter at the alleged times, Bruce would stick to his position, saying that her alibis were part of the conspiracy to cover her tracks. He told the therapist that he was an expert at secrets. Several years previously, he had found out that his sister was actually his mother, who had been inpregnated by his father when she was 14. Bruce felt that if he could uncover that story, nothing could stop him from ferreting out any sort of secret.

The Heart's relationship to the mind is reflected in sleep patterns, as well. People with imbalances in Fire show a variety of sleep disruptions. Night should be a time for *yin*, a period when the body and mind can rest and restore. Insomnia is generally produced by an imbalance between *yin* and *yang* that prevents the transition from the activity of day to the quiet of night. Problems with falling asleep are usually caused by a deficiency of Heart *xue*, the lack of nourishment to the mind preventing it from entering a quiet state. If one can fall asleep but wakes during the night, the insomnia is generally created by a deficiency of Heart *yin*, the relative preponderance of *yang* activity being sufficient to rouse one from the sleep state. Insomnia accompanied by a restless mind or sleep that is disrupted by vivid dreams is generally produced by an excess of heat in the Heart.

The Heart also contains and maintains a person's *shen*. Remember that *shen* is the essence of character, one's spirit and sparkle. If the Heart is functioning adequately, *shen* shines in one's face and eyes; there are warmth and vitality, aspirations and compassion. If the Heart is deficient or blocked, the spirit is poor, the eyes don't shine, and recovery is difficult. Clients can also present with false *shen*, an appearance of vitality masking an underlying serious deficiency, as seen in those who work hard to present a positive façade despite severe underlying problems. The illusions created by some psychopathic clients are another example of false *shen*.

Angie, a 32-year-old psychologist, was seen as the guru of the therapeutic community in her small town. She ran a successful therapy clinic and was often consulted by both community agencies and other therapists for help with difficult cases. Angie had been married for 10 years to Jack, and they had two children. Her appearance was that of a confident, well-adjusted pillar of society.

At a meeting with some colleagues, Angie broke the news that she was making major changes in her life. She said that she had decided to attend medical school in another state, since she felt she could accomplish more as a psychiatrist. Angie had moved out of her house and into a rented one on the same street, in preparation for the larger move out of town, so that her family could adjust to the separation. Several days later, one of the attendees bumped into Angie and her husband. When he commiserated with Jack about the impending changes, Jack looked confused, and Angie quickly changed the subject. Further investigation by other colleagues revealed that Angie had never moved out of her house, was not going to medical school, and, in fact, had a master's degree in social work, not a doctorate in psychology. Her title of "Dr." came from a degree in fine arts.

Fire is related to the tongue, not in its eating role, which is an Earth function, but as it pertains to speech. The fluidity of speaking is a Heart process, and the health of the organ determines whether there is stammer or a good connection to thought processes. Clients who hesitate when speaking or who can't find the right words to express themselves might have a Fire imbalance. Being "tongue-tied" or "loose with the tongue" is indicative of Fire difficulties. Both garrulous speech and elective mutism can be connected to an imbalance in this element.

Pauly, six years old, was referred for therapy by his school. The boy would not speak in class, either to his teacher or to the other students. When the school contacted his parents, they refused to believe this, stating that Pauly talked continually at home. He had never attended kindergarten or preschool programs, but there were no signs that his reluctance to speak could be attributed to apprehension or anxiety at being away from home. Pauly did all of his work and played readily with other children; he just wouldn't speak. When he showed up for school one day with severe bruises, a social worker was contacted. It was determined that there was abuse in the home. Pauly's silence had been the product of an admonition from his parents "never to say a word in school" about the family situation. He had taken the instruction to mean that he was never to talk in class at all.

Fire's connection to speech is also evident in a diagnostic pattern known as "phlegm misting the heart." This can be seen in manifestations of excess cold as well as of excess heat, both of which are serious conditions. The syndrome is the result of mental depression that causes *qi* to stagnate. The lack of energy flow means that fluids cannot circulate well, and the prolonged accumulation of fluids eventually congeals them into a thick phlegm. If there is also a lack of *yang*, the phlegm condition stays "cold." Symptoms first present as mental dullness or depression, as the phlegm begins to obstruct the mind, and speech becomes incoherent and unconnected. If the condition continues, it can result in catatonia or coma.

In the hot-phlegm aspect of the syndrome, the obstruction caused by the accumulation of fluids creates heat (like damming up a river to generate electricity). The mind becomes disturbed and the thoughts deranged. Sleep is disrupted by wild dreams, and there can be aggressive or violent behavior. Speech becomes incoherent and manic. Breathing is ragged and coarse.

Chantelle, a seven-year-old girl attending a school for emotionally disturbed children, began acting strangely in class. She started grunting louder and louder, increasing the volume of her outbursts despite requests from the teacher to stop. When the teacher approached her, Chantelle overturned her desk and started racing around the room, shrieking and pulling at her clothing. She was removed to the nurse's office with difficulty, writhing in the teacher's arms on the way. When she saw the cot in the nurse's room, Chantelle's hysteria increased. She began babbling incoherently, punctuating her utterances with "no, no." By the time the psychologist arrived, Chantelle had ripped off her clothes, screaming that snakes from the cot were crawling all over her body. The psychologist was able to calm Chantelle slightly by offering her a "magic" blanket to wrap around herself, one that would protect her from the snakes.

Fire rules over the blood vessels, which is not surprising given the element's relation to the Heart. Poor circulation is connected to Fire, and individuals with excessive cold in the element generally have chilly hands and feet. If a deficiency of Heart *yin* is creating a false-heat situation, the palms of the hand and the soles of the feet become very hot and sweaty. Since this is not a true excess-heat condition, the rest of the body feels dry owing to the deficient *yin* moisture, and it maintains a cool or normal temperature.

Palpitations frequently occur in relation to Fire problems, in part due to its connection with blood circulation. If *qi* is insufficient to drive the blood, palpitations arise because the blood can't move through the vessels smoothly. A deficiency of *xue* can also lead to palpitations since there is not adequate blood to nourish the Heart or promote its smooth functioning. They may also be experienced in excess conditions, such as stagnation of *xue* in the heart. This is the situation with a heart attack, when blood congeals in the vessels or the heart, preventing a smooth flow of *xue*. Palpitations also may be associated with excess heat in the Heart, since the increased temperature causes the blood to "boil," impeding smooth circulation. It is essential, then, that if a client reports palpitations as a symptom, a thorough differential diagnosis be conducted so that correct treatment can be planned.

Heat and summer are the climatic factor and season related to Fire. An excess of heat can disrupt the *shen*, make the mind manic, and disturb sleep. Individuals who have problems with the element often find their symptoms exacerbated in the summer or when they are exposed to excessive heat. Alcohol and cigarettes often create an excess of heat in the body and disrupt heart functioning. Cocaine destroys the *yin* aspect of the Heart and can create a false-heat effect, leading to alterations in memory, speech, and sleep. As sedatives consume Heart *yang*, thinking can be cloudy or muddled and *shen* suppressed when one is on these drugs.

Joy is the emotion associated with Fire and laughter the sound. When the element is functioning well, the person takes delight in work and family, and has a lilt to the voice and a sparkle in the eyes. When Fire is imbalanced, however, a variety of manifestations can arise. A deficiency of the element leads to a lack of enjoyment and flat affect. Nothing is of interest or can provoke a smile. The client's eyes have a dull, glazed look, and the person rarely pursues either activities or relationships. Therapy with these clients can be frustrating since they are difficult to invest in the therapeutic process. To achieve success, the therapist needs to find a way to stimulate warmth or interest.

Raymond, age 24, and his parents came to therapy for help with his motivation. He had been diagnosed as schizophrenic several years earlier, but the mental health unit staff felt that his biggest problem was his habitual use of marijuana. Raymond lived with his parents and two brothers. His father and a brother ran a car repair shop from the house. His parents, James and Susan Morton, complained that Raymond refused to do any housework, to help in the shop, or to look for work in town. Instead, he stayed in his room or watched television all day.

At the same session, Raymond sat quietly with a blank, vacant look on his face. Efforts by the therapist to engage him in conversation were futile, as Raymond insisted he had nothing to say. Even attempts at discussing favorite television programs were dismissed. Any suggestions about improving the situation at home were countered by, "I can't" or "I don't want to do that," so the therapist shifted to a more indirect approach. Mr. Morton was asked to spend all of his time with Raymond, including sleeping in the same room. Raymond's brother would handle more responsibility in the repair shop, and his mother would assist with paperwork to free up her husband's time. The suggestion provoked a response from Raymond. He vehemently insisted that he didn't want his father intruding in his life. Mr. Morton also protested, saying that he couldn't meet his work obligations while baby-sitting his son all day. With some prompting from the therapist, however, Mr. Morton eventually agreed to the plan.

Raymond was forced to stop smoking marijuana because of his father's continual presence. After several weeks of the intervention, he found work in town so that he could escape his father's company. They did, however, continue eating dinner together, and Mr. Morton would go into Raymond's room in the evening to watch television. Raymond confided to the therapist that he planned to keep his job because he preferred his father's company in small doses.

It is hard to conceive of an excess of joy or laughter, but it does happen. Clients who laugh inappropriately or uncontrollably are showing an excess of Fire. Excessive joy often manifests as mania or hysteria. Clients with an excess of heat in the Heart often rush around, darting from one project to another, full of misplaced enthusiasm. These manic phases can shift from excessive exuberance to irritation, eventually flaring up into aggression. Clients with true-heat mania often have red faces, rapid pulses, and a high level of thirst since the excess fire is boiling the blood and drying them out.

A false-heat mania, attributable to a deficiency of Heart *yin*, can also be observed. Clients in this state are not nearly as agitated, and have flushed cheeks rather than a red face, poor memory (since the *yin* is not nourishing the mind), hot palms and soles, and spontaneous night sweats. False-heat manics are the most likely to be diagnosed as bipolar since their manic state is the result of an inherent deficiency. When the relative heat predominates, the client is active and manic. When the underlying deficiency is prevalent, the client is subdued owing to the lack of nourishing essence. Therapies for true-heat mania and false-heat mania would be radically different. Treatment for false-heat mania requires providing the client with nurturance, warmth, and support to supplement the deficiency. The true-heat condition would benefit from therapy that redirects the activity into more appropriate directions, eventually reducing the excess levels.

Doris, 39 years old, was referred for therapy by her doctor because of concerns about her behavior. Dr. Clement said that the family maintained that Doris would compulsively spend the household income. On a more personal level, he said that she would talk nonstop while being examined and become extremely flirtatious. Doris came to the first session with her husband, Richard. According to background information, the couple had two daughters—Julie, 18, who was in her first year at college; and Christine, 16, who spent her free time with her boyfriend. Richard said Doris was devoted to the children and had developed her strange behavior after they had grown up and found their own interests. Doris, an accomplished musician, used to love to play the piano while the two girls accompanied her on other instruments.

Doris complained that she was unable to concentrate on anything for very long, jumping from one activity to another. If she didn't achieve success on a project quickly, she became irritable. Richard would encourage her to settle down to one activity, hoping this would decrease her frustration, but his efforts were futile. The therapist decided to use Doris' musical inclinations and interest in the children to help solve the problem. Christine was asked to play music with her mother for an hour each evening. Richard would record the sessions, and the family would decide which tape to send to Julie each week, along with messages telling her how much they missed her. Everyone in the family liked the idea. Doris would practice during the day instead of shopping, so that the recording would be special. Richard loved seeing his wife more focused. Christine grudgingly agreed to the plan as it only took one hour of her time each night, and it made her feel more connected to her sister. Julie started sending back tapes of her own guitar solos, which the family would listen to in the evenings. Gradually, the recording sessions decreased to once or twice a week, as Doris began playing with a community orchestra.

Panic attacks are another manifestation of either excess or deficiency in the Heart. True-heat conditions are characterized by a flushed face, marked restlessness, palpitations, severe anxiety, insomnia with active dreaming, a racing mind, and a rapid pulse. In false-heat panic attacks, the person experiences vague restlessness, palpitations, blurring of vision and thinking, sweaty palms and soles of the feet, and an inability to fall asleep at night. True-heat panic attacks are the result of excess heat in the Heart, whereas the false-heat panic reactions are a product of insufficient cooling *yin* energy in the organ.

Red is the color associated with the element. The taste related to Fire is bitter, as in horseradish, unsweetened chocolate, or coffee. Clients with cravings for bitter foods or who have a bitterness toward life could be demonstrating a Fire imbalance. Logically, a burnt or scorched smell is associated with the element. Patients in the last throes of a debilitating illness often emit a burnt smell when their heart begins failing. Dreams of fire or scorched earth can be indicative of an imbalance in the element.

Fire depression is highlighted by joylessness and sleeping difficulties. The client shows little spirit or affect. Even the most humorous events or stimuli can't provoke a smile. The person has difficulties in speaking or expressing his or her thoughts. Memory and thinking are impaired. There can be panic attacks or shifts into mania. Suicides involve slashing the arteries, particularly those in the wrists.

## CHAPTER THIRTEEN

### The Law of Five Elements

■

*So sometimes things are ahead and sometimes they are behind;*
*Sometimes breathing is hard, sometimes it comes easily;*
*Sometimes there is strength and sometimes weakness;*
*Sometimes one is up and sometimes down.*
*Therefore the sage avoids extremes, excesses, and complacency.*

—*Lao-tzu*

By looking at each of the five elements independently, a practitioner can make an assessment as to where the principal imbalances lie within a client. Table 13.1 summarizes aspects of the five elements that assist in the diagnostic process. Most people have a particular element that dominates their symptomatology. When exposed to a disruptive life event, Earth individuals might incur eating and digestive problems, become ruminative, or develop obsessions, whereas in the same circumstance, Water types might display anxiety, phobias, or sexual dysfunction. Acute events that are sufficiently powerful or prolonged can override constitutional tendencies, so that a Metal type might develop the Wood symptoms of migraines or anger if continually frustrated and hampered by obstacles.

In reality, difficulties rarely arise in a single element, but usually become manifest as an interplay or imbalance among several of them. For therapy to be effective, one needs to identify the relative excesses and deficiencies of each element and evaluate how they can be used to address the client's issues.

Within the Eastern healing framework there is a model that describes

| | Wood | Fire | Earth | Metal | Water |
|---|---|---|---|---|---|
| **Color** | Green | Red | Yellow | White | Black |
| **Season** | Spring | Summer | Change | Autumn | Winter |
| **Sense organ** | Eyes/vision | Tongue/ speech | Mouth/taste | Nose/smell | Ears/hearing |
| **Tissue** | Muscles and tendons | Blood vessels | Flesh | Skin | Bones |
| **Climate** | Wind | Heat | Damp | Dryness | Cold |
| **Process** | Birth | Growth | Transformation | Harvest/ maturation | Storage |
| **Emotion** | Anger | Joy | Contemplation | Grief | Fear |
| **Sound** | Shouting | Laughing | Singing | Whining | Groaning |
| **Flavor** | Sour | Bitter | Sweet | Pungent | Salty |
| **Smell** | Rancid | Scorched | Cloying | Rotten | Putrid |
| **Dreams** | Fatigue, wood, mushrooms | Fire, burning | Food, home, walls | Flying, cruel killing | Water, ships |
| **Function** | Move *qi* | Provide warmth, move blood | Transform and transport | Make *qi*, eliminate waste | Cool and moisten |
| **Spiritual aspect** | Soul, decision making | *Shen*, spirit | Thought | Instinct | Will |
| **Organs** | Liver and Gall bladder | Heart, Pericardium, Small Intestine, and Triple heater | Spleen and Stomach | Lung and Large intestine | Kidney and Bladder |

**Table 13.1.** *The Five Elements and Their Corresponding Characteristics*

these systemic connections—the Law of Five Elements. The law (diagrammed in Figure 13.1) details the relationships among Earth, Metal, Water, Wood, and Fire in both optimal and disease states. As in most of the underlying philosophies of Eastern medicine, the law is congruent with events in the environment; the description of what happens in the individual parallels cycles that occur in nature itself.

There are two basic patterns found among the elements. The first cycle is the promotional sequence that describes the process of creation and growth. It is represented by the dashed lines in Figure 13.1. In this cycle, each element creates the one that follows. As in nature, wood is used to generate fire, the ashes of fire create earth, the distillation of earth produces metal, the components of metal (remember that this element is also known as air) compose water, and water is used to make

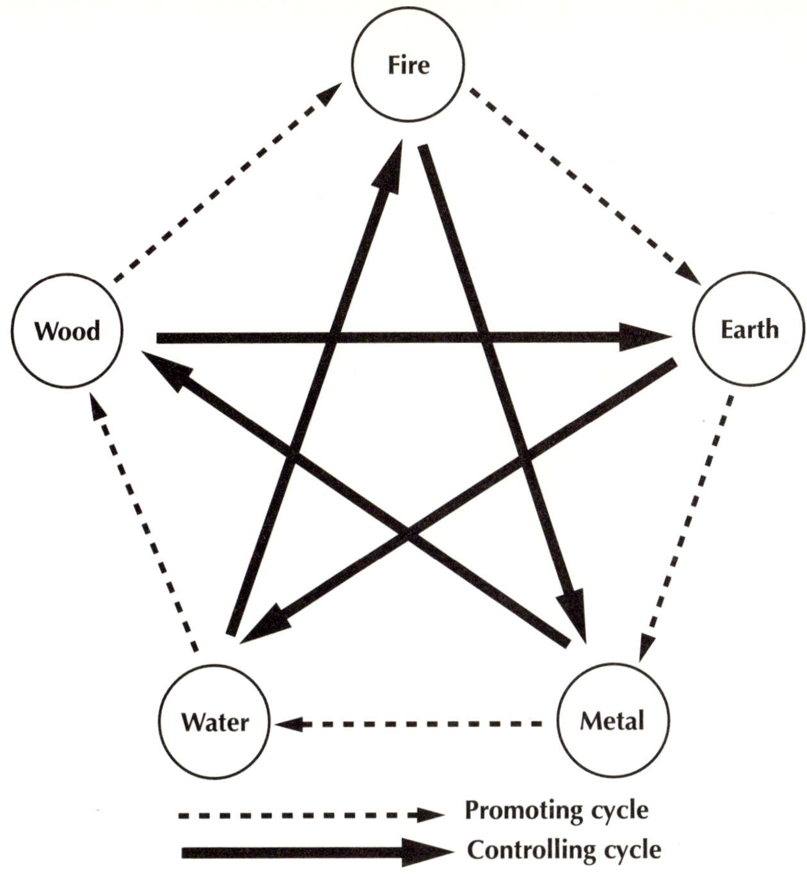


**Figure 13.1.** *The Law of Five Elements.*

wood grow. The direction of the cycle is critical to well-being. If flow is in the appropriate direction, the system is healthy. If the pattern reverses itself, however, disaster occurs—fire burns and consumes wood, wood dams up the free flow of water, water causes metal to rust, metal decreases the earth's fertility, and earth damps out fire. Effective treatment depends on promoting changes in the appropriate direction.

The pattern can be illustrated using emotions. Obviously, health results when an individual expresses emotions suitable to environmental events at appropriate levels. When emotions become stuck, however, it is usually because an imbalance is present. According to the Law of Five Elements, the natural transition of emotions should be from joy to contemplation, contemplation to grief, grief to fear, fear to anger, and anger to joy. Therapy that moves feelings in this direction would be more likely to restore healthy functioning. A client who is violent and aggressive could be asked to spend time watching funny movies or engaging in pleasurable activities. Clients who are fearful or anxious could be encouraged to express displeasure at an appropriate target. Although the situation is generally more complex than this even in the Eastern framework, the Law of Five Elements provides a model for treatment that might be beneficial and warns about movement against the flow. For example, clients who are grieving often shift into major depression if their sadness becomes rumination. Therefore, therapy that is action oriented might be more successful with sad clients than one that encourages them to contemplate their problems.

There is also an interfacing between the Law of Five Elements and the Eight Principles system. Difficulties arise if the "mother" element, the one that precedes another, is either excessive or deficient. Too much water would flood the root system of a tree, creating rot and stagnation, whereas an insufficient amount of moisture would cause the tree to wither and die. Problems of excess or deficiency not only affect the element concerned, but also can create a domino effect along the cycle.

Paul presented for therapy depressed and overweight. He said that all he cared to do lately was sit at home, eat, and watch television. When questioned about whether this was typical behavior for him, Paul said that a year earlier he had been quite driven. He had pushed hard in business and was quite a "ladies' man." He said that it had not been uncommon for him to end a long day at the office by drinking at a bar and going home with someone he barely knew. At some point, that lifestyle had begun to take its toll. Paul found himself feeling irritable and without the same sense of drive. He began to snap at colleagues and was abusive to women, as well. He gradually found himself losing interest in everything. Paul developed problems with sleep and experienced palpitations. His doctor suggested that he take some time off, but the two weeks of rest stretched into two months, as Paul isolated himself in his house and ate himself into his present size. He couldn't stand the person he had become, but he didn't seem to have the energy to do anything about it.

Paul's frantic lifestyle had consumed vital essence, *jing*, and produced a deficiency of Water energetics. The decreased level of Water energy meant that the next element, Wood, was not sufficiently cooled or nourished. Paul's temper flared and he experienced the fits and starts of a nonflowing Liver system. In turn, Wood became incapable of generating enough Fire energy, resulting in sleeping problems, palpitations, and a lack of joy. The diminished Fire caused an Earth deficiency, producing isolation in the home, rumination, and an attempt to restore energetic levels by increasing food intake. The overconsumption of food in Paul's deficient state, however, created a further stagnation and an inability to provide the Metal element with the proper nourishment to generate *qi*. What began as a disruption of a single element created ramifications throughout the entire system.

The promotional cycle is only one aspect of the Law of Five Elements. For balance, there has to be a mechanism of control, as well as of generation, or growth would proceed unchecked. The control cycle, illustrated by the solid lines in Figure 13.1, describes the pattern of restraint that the elements place on each other. As in nature, Wood checks Earth by preventing erosion, Earth slows down the movement of Water, Water cools raging Fire, Fire melts and shapes Metal, and Metal cuts Wood down to size. Again, for the cycle to work effectively, the flow must occur in the prescribed direction, and no element should overpower another. If one element exerts too much control, it creates problems in the recipient in the same way that an overpowering spouse causes shifts in the other spouse's behavior. Water can keep Fire under control, but a dousing puts it out.

If one considers the emotional aspect of the control cycle, some helpful guidelines emerge. Wood, and its associated emotion of anger, is controlled by Metal, sadness. This suggests that aggression can be modulated by remorse, a technique frequently used in anger-management programs. The anger of Wood can be used to temper Earth's excessive contemplation. Clients who are mired in thought patterns can often be moved out of them by encouraging action and movement. The thinking processes of Earth are used to control the fear aspect of Water, which may be the reason why Cognitive Behavior Therapy achieves such success with phobias and anxiety. Water controls the excessive joy of Fire, in that apprehension of consequences can mitigate unrestrained manic behavior. Finally, the joy of Fire can chase the grief and sadness of Metal, as in the mourner who finds a reason to live in the smile of a grandchild.

In the remainder of this chapter, the Law of Five Elements will be applied to individual therapy cases, and in the next chapter, the use of the system in interpersonal situations will be addressed.

## Illustrative Cases

### *Jeremy*

Jeremy, a 41-year-old jazz musician, presented for therapy at the recommendation of his physician. He was having problems with cluster headaches that seemed unresponsive to any standard medical treatment. Changes in diet, massage, and pharmaceuticals produced little change in his symptoms. Jeremy was becoming irritable at not getting better, his mood not improved by the fact that the headaches usually started at 1 A.M. and kept him awake all night long.

Jeremy reported that he had previously experienced similar bouts of cluster headaches. This latest episode had begun after he had moved in with a woman, relocating from another city so that he could be with her. He said that he really cared for Trish, but was beginning to question whether the move was a good one. On some days, he felt that he wanted to settle down with Trish, even marry her, and on other days, he thought he should move out. Jeremy stated that his decision to live with Trish was quite impulsive, as they had only known each other for a month. In fact, at the time he met Trish, Jeremy had already committed to moving to Detroit to be with a woman he had met during a club engagement there. He was surprised at how angry the woman had become when he told her that he had met someone else. Jeremy had married at the age of 19, but the marriage only lasted three months. He had considered canceling the wedding right before the ceremony, but he was concerned about disappointing his relatives. Since then, he had been engaged at least three other times but never actually married again.

Jeremy said that his success with women was beyond his understanding, since he frequently had difficulty obtaining an erection, especially during the early stages of a relationship. He felt that his problem was due to insecurity about the size of his penis, fearing that women would ridicule him, and so he usually put off sex until they were hooked on him emotionally. He said that he sometimes used his bad back as an excuse to delay intimacy.

Jeremy also expressed irritation at his parents, who had never been supportive of his musical career, and it made him angry to think of how hard he had to struggle because they hadn't given him the background his talent deserved. He loved and respected them, but he felt that no matter what he did, he just couldn't please them. He vacillated between running home to see them and ignoring them for extended periods of time. Even when Jeremy was excited about a visit with his parents, he usually charged out of the house soon after getting there.

Jeremy's problem is produced by excess heat in Wood caused by an underlying Water deficiency, indicated by his sexual problems and lower back pain. Because Water is the mother of Wood, a deficiency in this element creates a situation in which Jeremy's Wood energetics are not sufficiently cooled or nourished. Both decision making and commitment depend on the smooth functioning of Wood. Jeremy's waffling and impulsive responses reflect the underlying deficiencies at the core of this element. In addition, because Water is not serving its cooling function, the *yang* aspects of the son element, Wood, begin to flare up. Jeremy's irritability and cluster headaches are the result of Wood's heat rising because of the absence of a grounding *yin* component. (Figure 13.2)

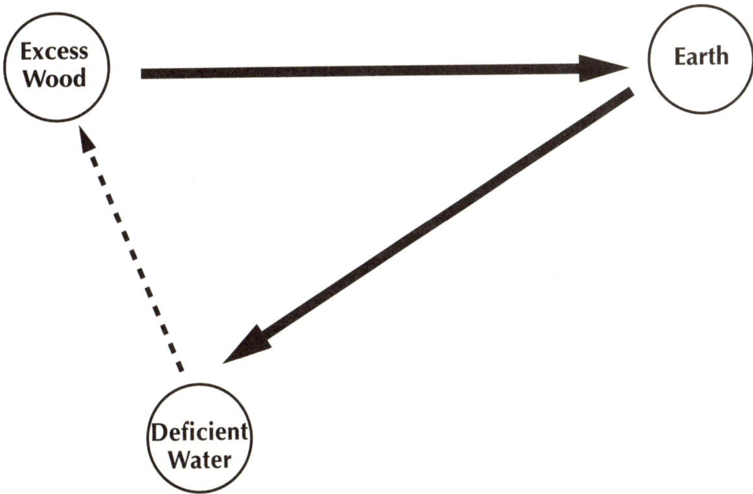


**Figure 13.2.** *Jeremy: deficient Water/excess Wood.*

Jeremy's treatment should focus on restoring his *yin* Water component while diffusing the heat accumulating in Wood. Earth, with its triangulated relationship to both elements via the control cycle, would be a logical choice for therapy. Increasing the *yin* components of Earth by increasing nourishing food and fostering a sense of home and family should improve Jeremy's deficient Water *yin*. Therapy that encouraged Jeremy to develop a constant relationship with his family instead of vacillating in his feelings would create a more solid Earth foundation, and also construct the basis for stabilizing his relationship with women. At the same time, Jeremy's *yang* Wood characteristics could be diffused toward the Fire element by having him channel the excess energy into something he likes, directing his pain and anger into joy. For example, every time Jeremy got a headache or became annoyed, he could spend 15 minutes playing his favorite tune or watching a movie (of course, given the fact that his symptoms often occurred in the early hours of the morning, this could also serve to bring his relationship with Trish to a head). If he were unable to function during the painful headache episodes, Jeremy could be asked to spend a certain amount of time engaging in pleasurable activities before going to sleep. Alternatively, meditation exercises, goal setting, and analytical planning could foster Jeremy's Earth energetics, simultaneously nourishing Water and pulling the excess heat out of the Wood element.

All of the suggestions could be unified in a single strategic intervention, such as proposing that Jeremy was not well enough to handle the stress of living with Trish. To improve, he would need to commit to returning home for at least six months and allowing his parents to care for him. His mother could cook nourishing meals, and his father could spend time listening to Jeremy practice his music. Jeremy could amuse himself by meditating and by helping out around the house.

### *Maggie*

Maggie, a 35-year-old mother of three, had left her husband after finding him with another woman. Maggie had been diagnosed by a series of psychiatrists as having borderline personality disorder, as well as problems with multiple personalities. She attended therapy because she was feeling suicidal and depressed. One of her seven personalities daily instructed her to kill herself. Other alters tried to mother her or ridicule her into good behavior. When the voice of the one personality became too strong, Maggie would attempt suicide, usually by trying to hang herself.

Maggie had been agoraphobic in the past, and she continued to be fearful of strangers. She also refused to have anything to do with her family of origin. She suspected her father of having sexually abused her when she was a child, and her mother had attempted to kill her with a knife shortly after Maggie got married. Her estrangement from her family became complete when her two sisters and her brother sided with her parents against her.

Maggie was highly intelligent, but she often distorted comments from others to mean that she was stupid, worthless, and ugly. She frequently became obsessed and enmeshed with people she did care about. As a result, she spent much of each day isolated at home, eating and worrying about the children, which didn't leave her much energy for doing anything else.

Maggie's difficulties appear to be manifesting in the Earth and Metal elements. Her Earth imbalance produces problems with thought processes, including a tendency to "flesh" out (an Earth-related metaphor) her disruptions into the form of multiple personalities. Maggie also ruminates, frequently linking this process to eating. Her Earth-based relationship problems are exacerbated by Metal difficulties, which create intense defensive barricades. This overactive protective energy shuts out most stimuli while walling in others, resulting in agoraphobia, detachment, and enmeshment. Maggie's intelligence often works against her by concocting elaborate mental scenarios and distorting information.

Although there is an excess of energy in Maggie's Earth element, that energy is not released to the son element, Metal. This leads to a lack of energy as *qi* cannot be produced. The imbalance also imbues her rumination with a sense of despair, often culminating in suicide attempts. Her attempts at hanging herself symbolize her trying to close herself off from the stimulation, air, and *qi* of the outside world. (Figure 13.3)

Therapy with Maggie needs, first of all, to encourage her to release some of the excessive Earth energy. This could be done by using her attachment to her children to hook her into establishing more adaptive boundaries, channeling some of the Earth energy into Metal along the promotion cycle. Maggie could be encouraged to attend meetings at school, allow her children to invite

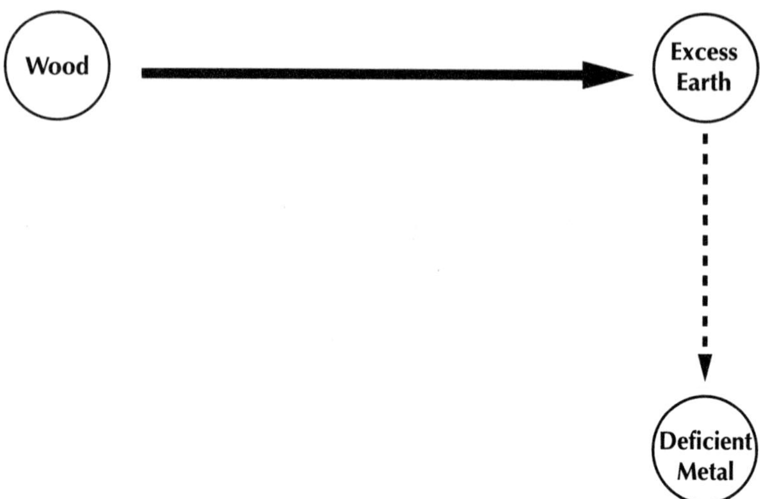


**Figure 13.3.** *Maggie: excess Earth/deficient Metal.*

friends to the house, and involve herself in their interests. The activity would also help shift some of the Earth-driven mental processes into a more active context, creating movement within the system. The control cycle could also be utilized to rein in some of Maggie's harmful thought processes. Wood functions, such as goal orientation and planning, could modulate some of her destructive thoughts and help her to reframe them. By establishing goals, such as obtaining a college degree so that she could better support her children, her intelligence could be utilized in a positive manner. Her multiple personalities could also be organized in the context of whether they were allowing her to achieve her necessary goals. An externalization of her alters might be achieved by transferring their qualities to actual people, moving the problem from an internal difficulty to an external one, thereby making it more accessible to treatment.

### *Adam*

Adam, a 26-year-old computer programmer, was diagnosed with paranoid schizophrenia. He lived with his mother, and was referred for therapy after intentionally setting fire to the couch. His mother explained that Adam first began having problems nine years earlier when she and his father separated. Adam had been very close to his father, despite the father's alcoholic rages. During the messy divorce, he had begun behaving in a very flamboyant manner, acting out or exposing himself in public. He frequently laughed inappropriately, as if someone were telling him a joke that only he could hear. He was a bright man and a hard worker, but he usually lost jobs by doing something bizarre in the office. He was most recently terminated because he stood on his desk shouting that he was a homosexual and daring anyone to say anything negative about it.

Adam said he often felt compelled to speak out. He lit the fire after his mother told him he needed to improve his behavior at work, adding that he got the inspiration for the act from a dream he had had the night before. He said that his dreams were very vivid and instructive, and that he often experienced them during the day, as well as at night. He said that he loved his mother and hadn't wanted to upset her, and he was afraid that she might be sufficiently annoyed this time to make him leave home. Adam was worried about this possibility, he said, because he wasn't sure he knew how to cook.

The separation of Adam's parents triggered a high level of anxiety and fear, depleting his Water energetics and leading to an inability of that element to regulate his Fire. Without the balancing coolness, Adam's Fire energies began to flare out of control. Joy, unrestrained, developed into hysterical and inappropriate laughter. The deficiency of Water also allowed him to act without fear of consequences. The heat in his Fire element agitated Adam's mental functioning, producing vivid dreaming and wild thoughts. As the Fire raged out of control, it further consumed any vestige of controlling *yin* Water elements, resulting in activity without any possibility of restraint. (Figure 13.4)

Therapy needs to focus on restoring Adam's balancing *yin* energies to cool the *yang* while directing some of his Fire energies into Earth. This could be achieved by telling Adam that his situation at home would depend on his ability to stay in a job. If he acted in an appropriate manner at work, his mother would cook for him. If he acted in a manner that caused him to be dismissed, he would have to care for himself. The intervention serves two functions. The increased awareness of consequences should help temper Adam's unrestrained behavior by directly improving his Water aspect. If he conducted himself properly at work, his comfort at home, an Earth component, would

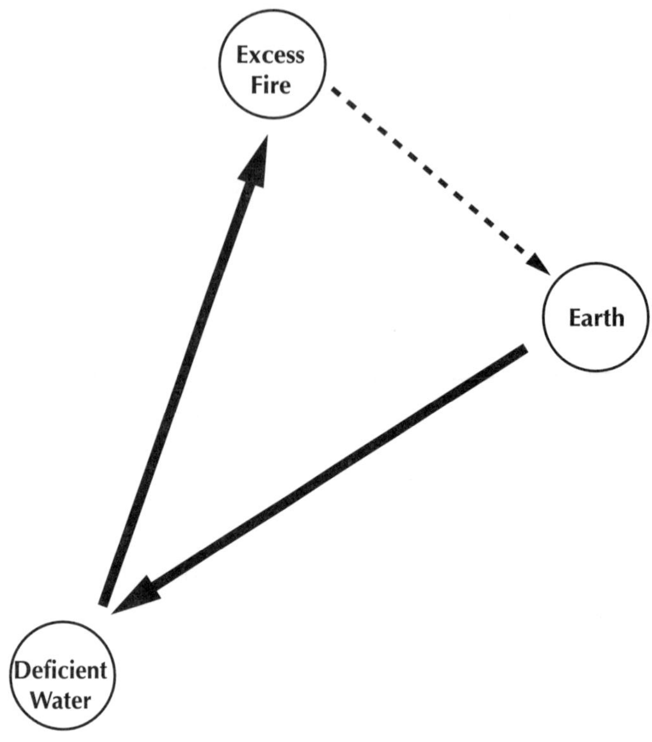


**Figure 13.4.** *Adam: deficient Water/excess Fire.*

feed into his Water energetics, ultimately fostering better control over his Fire. Additionally, Adam's excessive Fire would be drained into Earth, by directing him to become involved in home-based activities whenever his actions were out of control.

***Sarah***

Sarah, a 24-year-old graduate student, was first seen in the hospital as part of the collecting of evidence related to her being sexually assaulted. She had awakened one night to find a man on top of her, holding a knife to her throat. He threatened to kill her if she didn't follow his instructions. The assault had been brutal, and seemingly endless. By the time her assailant had removed the knife from her throat, Sarah didn't feel that she had the will to call for help. She lay dazed in bed for over an hour. Finally, she sat up and called the police. When they arrived a short time later, she struggled to walk to the door to let them in. Her speech was low and incoherent. An ambulance was called, and Sarah was admitted to the hospital for evidence collection and observation. The police officers and doctors found it difficult to obtain information as Sarah vacillated between laughing hysterically and muttering incomprehensibly, and she seemed unable to understand simple questions.

Sarah's initial reaction shows many aspects of the Fire element. Her situation is called "scattered *shen*" in Eastern medicine, the shock of the events making her spirit and energy bounce around like a pinball. Fire is the element related to *shen,* and also to speech, thinking, and memory. Sarah's inability either to recall events or to describe them was an aspect of her Fire disruption. The Eight Principles theory would suggest using *yin* qualities to control the fiery *yang* problems. Creating a "cool" situation by placing Sarah in a quiet room with a calming individual would help achieve this goal. Once she had stabilized, the transition from Fire to Earth could be achieved by surrounding her with nurturant people, familiar objects, and nourishing food. She should then be better able to recall events and contemplate what had occurred. (Figure 13.5A.)

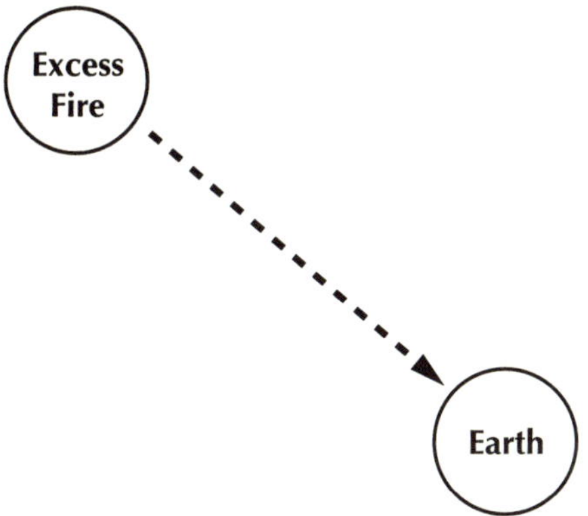


**Figure 13.5A.** *Sarah: excess Fire.*

Sarah presented for therapy a short time after her release from the hospital. Her appearance was radically different from her disheveled, distraught demeanor just after her assault. In fact, she was almost too neat and polished. Her speech was controlled as she described how well she was doing. She had resumed classes, made up her lost work, and installed new locks on her doors and windows. Sarah said she felt as though her biggest problem was that she didn't have enough energy to accomplish all she was trying to do. She also was unsure about whether she should go to her family's home for Christmas, not really wanting to rehash the events of the assault. Sarah had pulled away from most of her friends as well so that she wouldn't have to explain what had happened that night. She said she wasn't sure that therapy was a good idea at this time either, as she was doing fine and didn't want to be reminded of the assault. Sarah said she had attended this session only because it had been a condition of her release from the hospital.

Sarah's condition went from an external excess immediately following the trauma to an internal imbalance. Many of the aspects of her behavior were the result of the trauma's being pulled deep into the interior of her functioning where it could be walled off by protective energy, a function of the Metal element. This barrier allowed her to keep the incident out of her daily functioning, but it caused her also to defend against more benign influences, such as friends and family. Therapy could use the control cycle to temper Sarah's imbalance. By adding the warmth of the Fire element, such as encouraging her to have some fun with a supportive friend or family member and away from the assault issue, the strength of Sarah's barricade against beneficial outside influences might weaken. Alternatively, her detachment might be broken by causing her to become angry, either at the events that precipitated her assault or toward some other target, thus moving her energy from Metal to Wood. (Figure 13.5B)

Sarah returned to therapy when she began to experience difficulties with sleeping. She said that the slightest noise would awaken her, and she then would become worried that someone was in the house. Sarah had installed another set of locks, but they didn't reassure her. Her fears had begun to extend to daylight hours, and she reacted every time someone walked behind her or made a loud noise. A graduate student from another department had asked her out on a date, but Sarah didn't know whether she could trust him, and she couldn't stand the thought of a relationship that could lead to sex.

Sarah's problems have shifted into the element of Water, as evidenced by the high level of fear and the inability of Water to cool the mind during

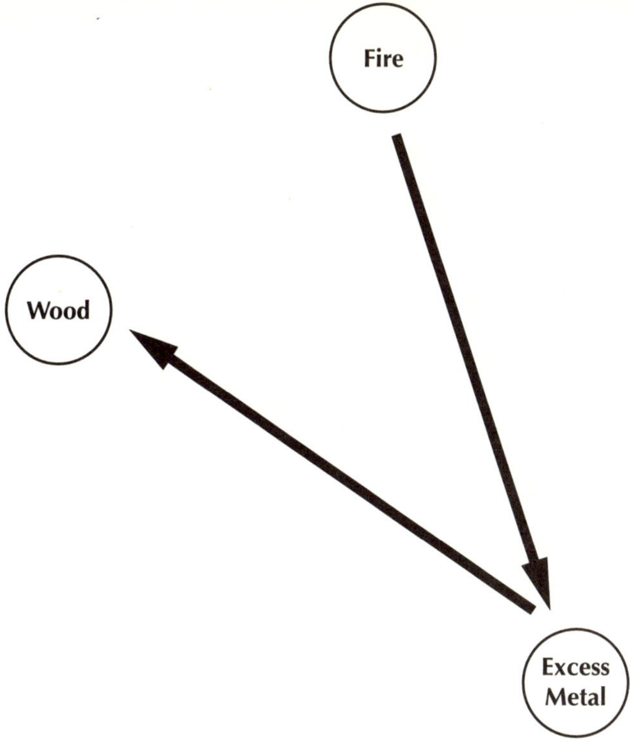


**Figure 13.5B.** *Sarah: excess Metal.*

sleep. Treatment could use either the promotional or control cycle to create change. Sarah could be encouraged to transform her fear into anger, beating pillows or writing a heated letter to her perpetrator, shifting the focus from Water to Wood. Alternatively, she could be encouraged to focus on things that gave her joy and pleasure, increasing these activities or associations whenever she became fearful, causing a transition from Water to Fire. The control cycle could also be utilized using the Earth element. Increasing her consumption of nourishing food, engaging in activities that would provide comfort, or using techniques to change her thought patterns could balance out Sarah's Water energetics by increasing the amount of controlling Earth influence. (Figure 13.5C)

All of the cases described show an interplay between underlying and presenting disharmonies. The Law of Five Elements allows for a systemic approach to both diagnosis and treatment. Patterns are defined

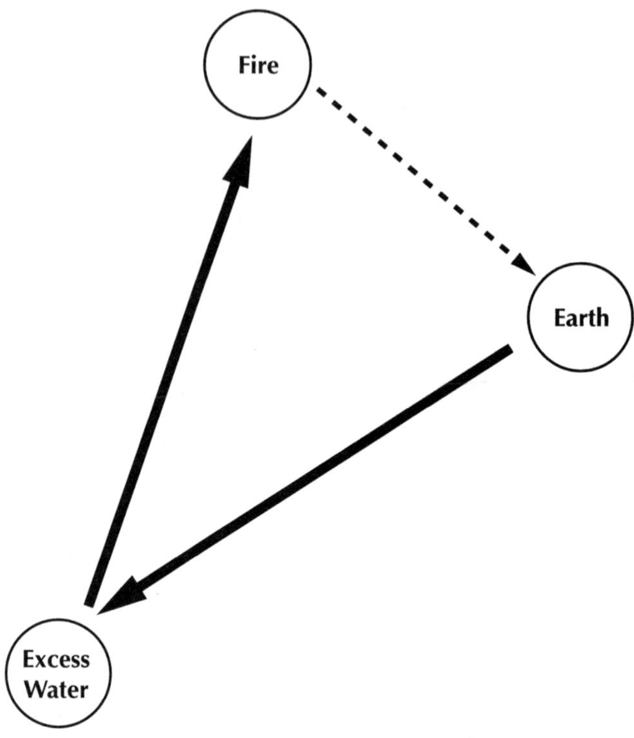


**Figure 13.5C.** *Sarah: excess Water.*

and a plan of action can be established. It is interesting to note that many of the difficulties assume a triangular pattern. In psychotherapy, the triad has frequently been used to describe interpersonal relationships, but rarely utilized to describe patterns within a person. In Eastern healing, even intrapersonal treatment is most effectively conceptualized using a three-point combination of the promotional and control cycles. In the following chapter, the model will be extended to interpersonal situations.

# CHAPTER FOURTEEN

## Interpersonal Five-Element Therapy

■

*Cultivate virtue in yourself,*
*And virtue will be real.*
*Cultivate it in the family,*
*And virtue will abound.*

—*Lao-tzu*

Eastern healing is, by nature, an individual affair. A patient presents for treatment, and the practitioner performs acupuncture, prescribes herbal formulas, or adjusts the person's diet. Although questions about the patient's family or lifestyle might be asked to ascertain background history, intervention is conducted on the individual. In psychotherapy, however, many modalities utilize an interpersonal approach. Whether in family therapy, systems work, psychodrama, or social action, treatment operates outside the boundaries of the identified client and the client's problems.

In this chapter, the Eastern healing perspective is extended to the context of interpersonal relations using the Law of Five Elements. Once again, the examples are not intended as a "how to," but rather as alternatives for those times when therapists find themselves stymied by a family and their difficulties, a perspective outside the norms of typical problem solving.

■

***Boswell Family***

The family presented for therapy after the suicide attempt of the son, Keith, a 17-year-old high school student. He had consumed a bottle of pills after being dumped by his girlfriend. An honor student and captain of the school soccer team, Keith was generally quiet and studious. He told the therapist that he had taken the pills because his girlfriend had abandoned him. They had dated since they were 13, and he now felt disoriented and alone. Keith had been depressed for two weeks prior to the suicide attempt, but he didn't tell his family. Whenever his mother asked why he wasn't eating, Keith would put her off, saying it was just a phase. He hadn't been able to concentrate well on his studies, spending all of his time rehashing the events before the breakup and trying to figure out what had gone wrong. When Keith realized that he hadn't completed a class project due the next day, he became even more despondent, feeling that his academic status was now in jeopardy. He took the pills because his problems were too overwhelming to hold inside any longer, and he couldn't think of any other way out.

Keith is showing many patterns of an Earth imbalance. His sense of abandonment and loss of place are aspects of that element, as are his decreased food intake and his tendency to ruminate. Attempted suicide by ingesting pills is also typical of Earth dysfunction. Keith's holding onto information and pain also suggests an inability of Earth to fulfill its function of transformation and transportation.

Keith's mother, Georgia, continually interrupted his responses. She alternated between interjecting comments about his girlfriend's being a worthless hussy and expressing anger at her son for attempting suicide, putting both his health and future at risk. When given a chance to talk, Georgia attacked everyone concerned. She held her husband, Vince, responsible for the suicide attempt, saying that it was his lack of involvement with Keith that allowed it to happen while she was at a club meeting. Georgia was even furious with the hospital staff members because they hadn't allowed her to stay with Keith while they worked with him, claiming that she was too disruptive. Georgia couldn't understand why her son hadn't approached her when he was feeling depressed, since she had helped him solve problems in the past.

> Georgia's behavior is suggestive of a Wood imbalance. Her anger and intrusive style suggest a high level of Wood *yang*. Even though she is clearly concerned about her son, she is unable to refrain from attacking him. Her Wood capability to plan and make decisions has been distorted into a tendency to control and dominate.

Vince, Keith's stepfather, sat impassively throughout his wife's tirade. When questioned by the therapist, he said he didn't feel that he had much to contribute. Vince said that he and Keith had always gotten along well, in part owing to their inherently quiet natures. He said that he liked peace when he came home from work, so he usually let Georgia have her way in the family. He generally was happy with her decisions, and he liked the order and structure her organizational skills provided. Vince believed in positive "family values"—work, church, and home—and didn't see much need to expand on the basics. His life consisted of doing his job, coming home to a cooked meal, and spending the evening reading a book or watching television. He rarely spent time with Keith, except when they watched sports programs together.

> Vince is also showing an Earth pattern. His rigid, moralistic thinking and desire to have things in their proper places are aspects of the Earth element. His lack of activity suggests a deficiency of Earth *yang*, as there is little energy directed toward transformation. Even the continual influence of Georgia's Wood volatility doesn't penetrate the structure of Vince's Earth stability, and he reframes her behavior in a way that doesn't require his responding.

The five-element pattern of the Boswell family is diagramed in Figure 14.1. Both of the men have primarily Earth element characteristics, whereas Georgia demonstrates a Wood aspect. Treatment could use a combination of the promoting and control cycles. First, Keith and Vince could both be directed toward the Metal aspect of functioning, to restore flow and also, ultimately, to help temper Georgia 's Wood. This could be accomplished by encouraging Keith to grieve for his past relationship by having a "funeral" for it. Vince could assist Keith in developing a protocol for

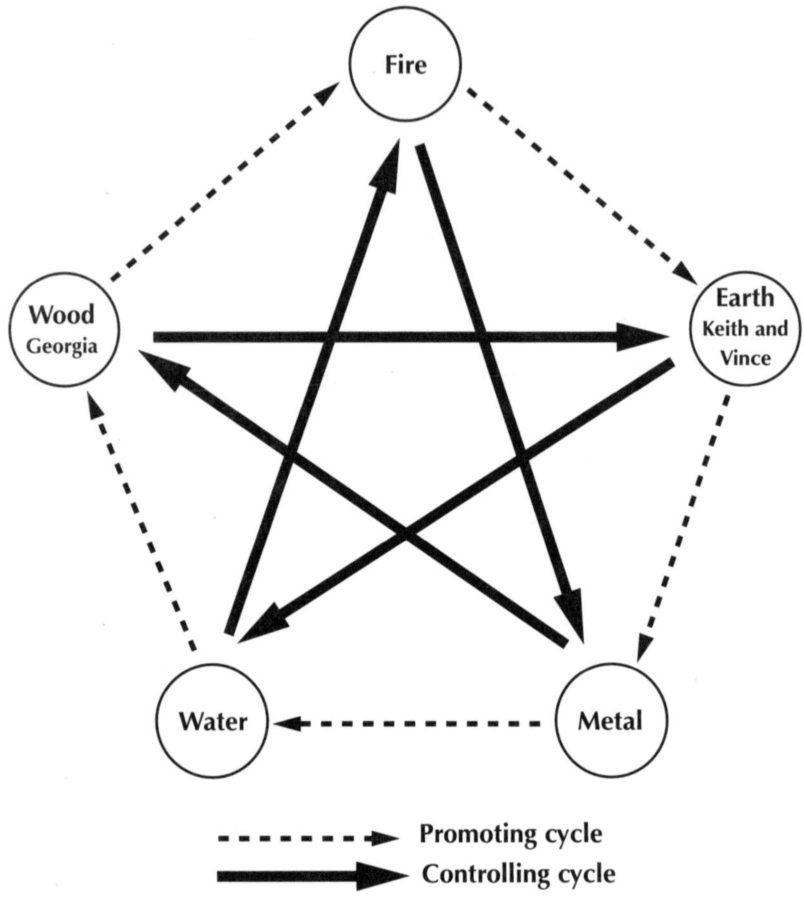


**Figure 14.1.** *Boswell family.*

the ritual, using Vince's moralistic tendency in a way that also promotes interaction and movement. The funeral would draw on the Metal functions of grieving and elimination by helping Keith move his stuck inner feelings to a more external level. The improved relationship between Keith and Vince should also help control the intrusion of Georgia 's Wood element.

Georgia should most likely be directed toward Fire to help draw off some of her excess Wood energetics. It could be suggested to her that she has been through an ordeal, above and beyond the high level of activity she normally expends for her family, so she deserves some pampering. She should be encouraged to spend a part of each day doing something that is either spiritually fulfilling or totally self-indulgent. Either choice would stimulate her Fire energetics, by increasing the *shen* or joy aspects, and would drain her excess Wood element in a beneficial manner. It is interesting to note that the intervention suggested by the Law of Five Elements is not very different from plans that might be developed in traditional family therapy where treatment might increase the involvement of the stepfather and son while refocusing the mother's attention to her own personal development.

***Hernandez Family***

The family presented for therapy at the recommendation of the school. Seven-year-old Carlos was often fearful in class, shying away from the teachers, as well as from other children. Even though the boy was usually a model student, he often would ask the teacher if he were going to be punished. Carlos said that voices inside his head were telling him he was bad. The worst of these voices belonged to the "Ta-ta Monster," who was mean and cruel and ready to pounce on Carlos at his slightest transgression. Carlos had very pale skin and dark circles under his eyes, and his voice was quiet, but deeper than might be expected. Whenever the boy's anxiety became overwhelming, he became incontinent. The enuresis never occurred at night because that was the time when the Ta-ta Monster patrolled, and Carlos was scared that the monster would find out if he wet his bed.

> Carlos is showing signs of a Water imbalance. This is manifest in his high level of fear and anxiety, his incontinence, and the dark circles under his eyes. The fact that Carlos' punishers take the form of voices might be related to Water's relationship to the sense of hearing. The deep quality of Carlos' voice is also similar to the groaning sound produced in Water imbalances.

Carlos' mother, Costanza, was gravely concerned about him, constantly praying for assistance with his problems. Costanza had tried various approaches—giving her son herbal remedies, sitting with him while he went to sleep, and talking to him about his problems—but nothing seemed to work. She loved her son dearly and wanted him to be well. Costanza thought that perhaps Carlos might do better if she schooled him at home, where he did not have to be so afraid. She had even considered talking to her priest about arranging an exorcism for Carlos, because she worried that the voices might be a sign of possession.

Costanza's main element appears to be Earth. She is highly nurturant and protective of her son. Her worry and concern are aspects of Earth's functioning, as are her attempts to transform the problem through succoring him and bringing him closer.

Carlos' father, Geraldo, seemed to find the whole situation absurd. He suggested that his son would be better served by punishing him than by indulging him. Geraldo was extremely disappointed that his only son was such a baby, as Carlos would run to his mother whenever his father came near him. The situation was exacerbated by the fact that Geraldo, almost choking with rage, would scream at Carlos whenever he ran away. Geraldo couldn't decide who was more ridiculous—his son, who allowed his mother to baby him, or the mother, who wouldn't let her boy grow up. Geraldo maintained that if he were allowed to deal with Carlos on his own terms, the difficulties would be resolved at once because he'd beat the voices out of the boy's head. Geraldo said he didn't believe in letting weaknesses rule your life. Whenever he got a severe headache, for example, he would immerse his whole head in cold water until the headache disappeared.

Geraldo's anger and aggression are suggestive of a Wood dysfunction. His tendency to shout and his violent headaches also suggest problems with that element. Geraldo's Wood attempts to control and penetrate Costanza's Earth element, but her intense need to protect Carlos repels the influence, causing Geraldo's levels of Wood energies to rise even higher.

The family dynamics are represented in Figure 14.2. Treatment might proceed in several directions. First, Carlos' energies could be pushed into the Wood element by transforming his fear into anger. This could be accomplished by having Geraldo become Carlos' protector against the voices in his head, particularly the Ta-ta Monster. Geraldo's anger and bravado could be channeled against the monster instead of against his son, making Carlos feel safe and uniting the father and child against a common target. Geraldo could be persuaded to do this by telling him that he needed to model for his son how to defend against enemies rather than run from them. By vanquishing the monster, Geraldo could show his son how a man behaves, and Carlos could learn to trust his

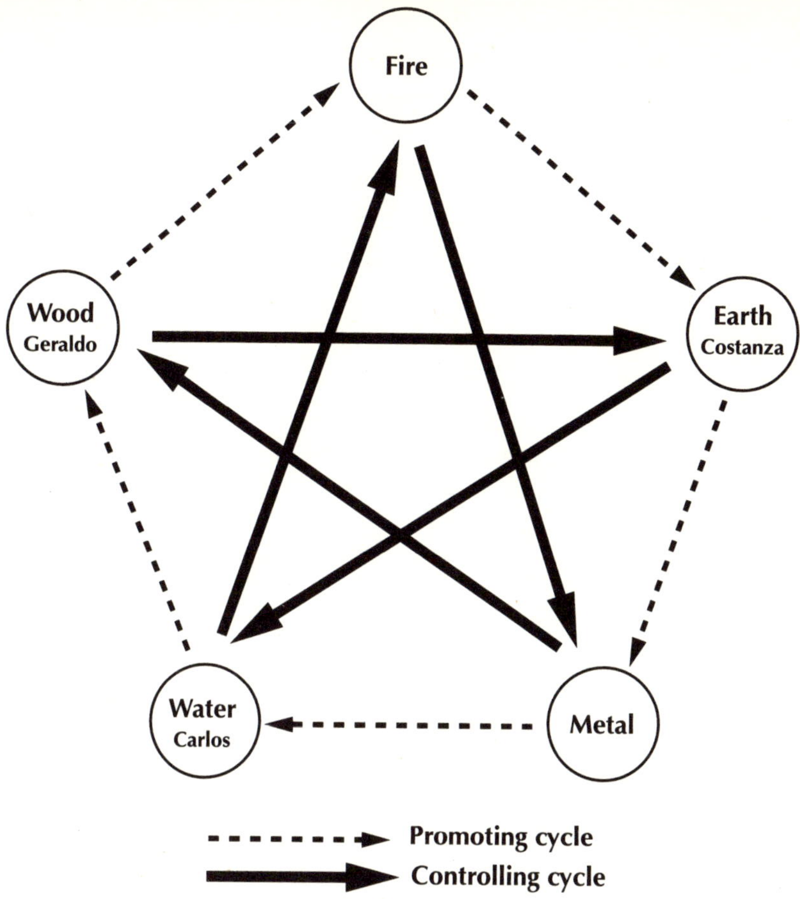


**Figure 14.2.** *Hernandez family.*

father rather than fear him.

The unification of father and son in a productive way in the Wood element should be sufficiently powerful to reduce the worrying in Costanza's Earth. Eventually, the father/son dyad should be moved to Fire, by encouraging them to spend time together doing pleasurable things, thus normalizing their relationship away from the fear issues.

***Philpott Family***

The family presented for therapy at the recommendation of a psychiatrist who had been treating nine-year-old Jared for ADHD. A few months earlier, Jared's father had committed suicide, and the boy's behavior had deteriorated significantly. In the session, Jared was extremely rude and belligerent, kicking over several chairs before sitting on the floor in the corner. He changed location frequently during the session, often by displacing other people from their seats. Jared wouldn't speak directly to the therapist, preferring to taunt other family members or to make rude noises while they were talking. His only other form of input was to make editorial comments, such as "dickhead" and "asshole," when certain people were mentioned.

Jared's behavior fits the category of excessive Wood heat, possibly caused by deficient Water or *yin* energy. His sudden outbursts and constant motion reflect the wind aspect of Wood disharmonies. His anger and inability to make good decisions are also indicative of problems in the Wood element.

Jared's mother, Amelia, was quite despondent and seemed almost oblivious to her son's outbursts. She said that she had previously been the supportive center of the family. When her husband shot himself over a failed business venture, Amelia seemed to have lost her focus as well. She spent most of the day in her room, either too sad or too tired to venture out. She spoke in a very low voice, a striking counterpoint to Jared's vocal interjections. In an even softer whisper directed toward the therapist, Amelia said that she was haunted by her husband's death. Some days, she said, she felt that the only way to block the memory from her awareness was by going blank, but that often caused her to forget to care for her children. If she had her way, Amelia said, she would prefer that everyone leave her alone so that she could rest, but there always seemed to be someone making a fuss. Amelia knew that things were falling apart, but she didn't have the strength to figure out what to do.

Amelia's primary problem seems to be in the Metal element, although indications are that she normally held an Earth function in the family. Metal is responsible both for producing *qi* and for creating protective barriers. Amelia's lack of energy, low voice, and desire to shut out the world are most likely related to a deficiency in the element. Metal is also associated with both grief and elimination. Amelia has not been able to effectively move out of her acute mourning and continually erects internal or external barriers to adaptive functioning.

Kerry, Amelia's seven-year-old daughter, seemed highly anxious, twisting and sucking on the tips of her long blond hair. Kerry agreed with anything the therapist suggested and was an easy target for manipulation by her brother. Amelia said that Kerry was making her crazy because the girl would not go into a room unless her mother or brother went in first to turn on the light and check the room out. Jared sometimes teased Kerry by pretending to make sure the room was safe, and then turning off the light as soon as she entered. Amelia said she had found Kerry huddled on the floor of her room one morning because Jared had told her that her father's ghost would get her in bed.

> Kerry's principal difficulties lie in the Water element, as she is extremely fearful and anxious. Kerry also shows deficient will, being unable to stand up to her brother or to force her mother to attend to her needs.

The session was also attended by Colin, the children's paternal uncle. Colin said that he was very distraught over his brother's death, and felt that the best way to handle his pain was to care for his brother's family. He also said that he was happily married, with two sons, one of whom got along fairly well with Jared. Colin worried about Amelia's ability to cope with the children and was concerned about Jared's out-of-control behavior and Kerry's fearfulness.

> Colin is best placed in the Earth element. He adds stability and nurturing to the situation. The Earth aspect is also reflected in his concern and worry about his brother's family.

The five-element pattern for the family is diagramed in Figure 14.3. An appropriate intervention might proceed in several directions. First, it could be recommended that Jared spend time with Colin and his family, moving his Wood energies toward a nurturant, better-centered Earth arena. Colin's strength and commitment, as well as his son's involvement, might drain some of the excess Wood heat found in Jared. The move would also help reduce Amelia's need to control her son so that she could concentrate on marshaling her own energies.

Amelia would probably benefit from initially concentrating on developing her own *qi* by feeding her deficient Metal aspect. This could be

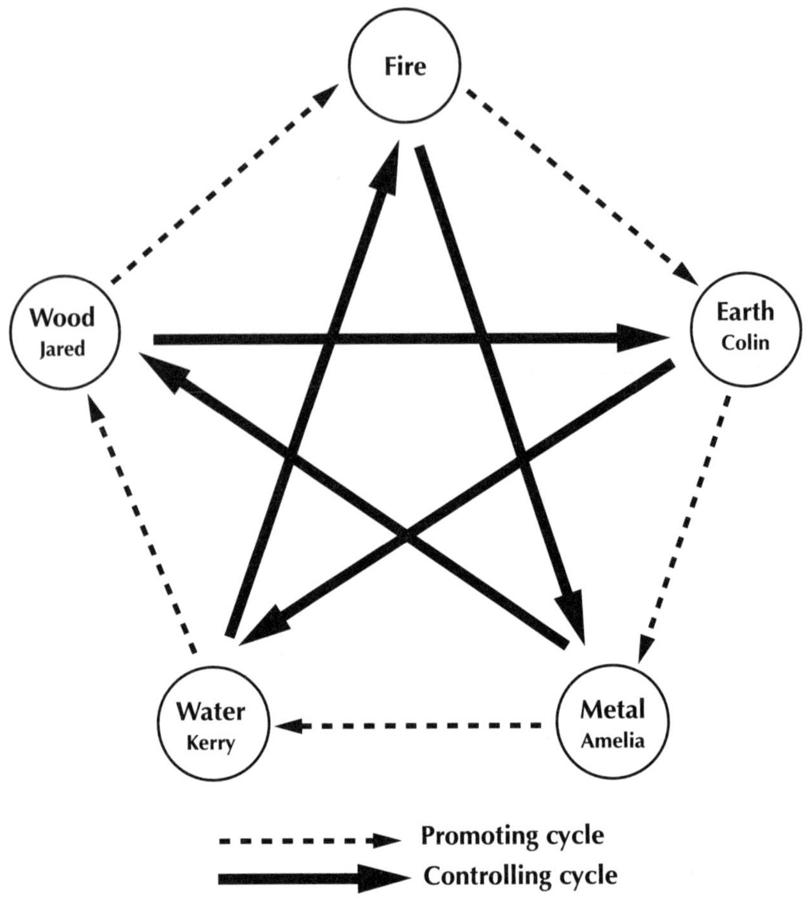


**Figure 14.3.** *Philpott family.*

accomplished by stimulating the mother element, Earth, through eating nourishing meals and increasing the comfort of her surroundings. Once Amelia has acquired sufficient energy, a factor that should be helped by not being continually drained by Jared's challenging behavior, she and Kerry could be encouraged to move toward the Wood element. Amelia would be helped by transferring grief into anger along the control cycle, while Kerry could transform her fear along the promotion cycle. Together, the pair could pound pillows or have shouting contests as a way of moving their energy. Amelia's renewed energy should also help reduce Kerry's fear since her mother would be acting more like herself.

■

***Edmond Family***

The family was referred for therapy by the father's psychiatrist. Max, a 32-year-old carpenter, had been diagnosed as bipolar about a year earlier. During his manic phases, Max would spend money recklessly, have affairs with other women, and work without sleeping. He became impulsive while driving, passing other cars with abandon and traveling at excessive speeds. Max's depressed moods made him listless and lethargic. He didn't want to do anything, including working or spending time with his children. He would sit huddled in his bathrobe for days, chain-smoking cigarettes. He sometimes drifted off to sleep during the day, but his nights were restless and fitful. Max was very charming during the session, although his answers were artfully crafted rather than direct, and he gave the impression of concealing more than he revealed. However, Max clearly cared about his family and missed them terribly.

Max is demonstrating two very different Fire patterns. His manic aspect is excess *yang*, raging Fire without any cooling component. This drives Max to act without any modulating consideration. His depressive behavior is a deficient *yang* manifestation. Once the Fire has burned itself out, Max is left with cold ashes. His lack of interest and joy and his inability to move are evidence of his lack of *yang*. Max cycles from one aspect to the other—the Fire builds, rages out of control, and then burns itself out. His clever speech and convoluted thinking are both related to the Fire element, which governs the mind and speech.

Nora, Max's wife, originally alternated between concern for Max and disgust over his behavior. After he had an affair with her sister, Nora lost most of her compassion, and the couple separated. She was against Max's having any contact with the children since he might either behave in a dangerous fashion or neglect them. Nora said that she was in charge of the family now, not Max, and it was up to her to decide what was in the best interest of the children. When Max came for a visit the week before, Nora lost her temper when he suggested that he take the kids out for some ice cream. They had a violent argument that ended when Nora threw a book at Max and ordered him out of the house. She understood that Max had a problem, but Nora could no longer ignore her anger toward him.

Nora is clearly operating in the Wood element. Her anger and shouting are one indication of this, but so is her planning for the family. While Nora might have originally held aspects of Earth and Fire that moderated her response to Max, his continual disruptive behavior has eliminated her other elemental influences.

The couple's nine-year-old son, Cory, presents as the most distressed member of the family. Cory generally had been a well-behaved boy, but his behavior had deteriorated considerably since the separation. He would cry over the slightest incident and whine whenever he didn't get what he wanted. Cory had stopped playing with his friends after school and sometimes wouldn't come out of his room even to watch TV. When Cory got sufficiently distressed, his bowels would become impacted. Cory said that he missed his father terribly. While Max frightened him sometimes, Cory liked it better when his father was around.

Cory is primarily showing aspects of the Metal element. He grieves for the loss of his father, and his sadness extends to the Large Intestine, a Metal organ. The sound of whining is also related to Metal, and Cory's erection of barricades against the outside world is a product of Metal's protective function.

Brad, the 12-year-old son, continually tried to set matters right between his family members. A considerate boy, he alternated between placating his mother, consoling his brother, and encouraging his father. Brad had frequently taken care of his father during his depressive episodes, trying to get him to eat something or attempting to cajole him out of the mood. He worried about who was going to do those things while his father was away from the family. Brad also comforted his mother when she became distressed over Max's actions, and he took a large part of the responsibility for running the household when no one else was capable. Brad was very concerned about his brother and was willing to do whatever he could to help.

Brad is clearly falling within the Earth element. He is nurturant and concerned. Brad's worrying is an aspect of Earth, as is his need to bring order into the family. He has clearly assumed the Earth position of central figure around which everything else revolves. Brad is the most stable of the family members and the most likely to work toward transformation of their problems.

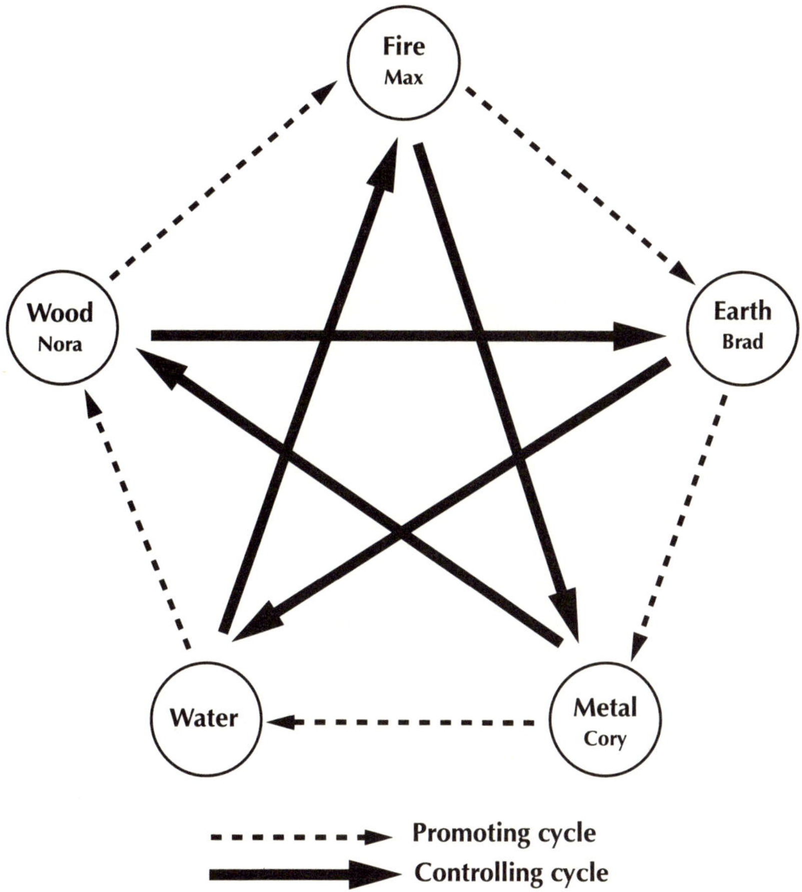


**Figure 14.4.** *Edmond family.*

Figure 14.4 illustrates the positions of the family members. Since Brad is the most centered and cooperative member of the family, it is probably best for any intervention to start with him. It could be suggested that he move into the Metal element with Cory, having him grieve with his brother over the loss of their father. This would "feed" into Cory's deficient Metal energy, but also would help to replace Max somewhat with an older brother. Nora should be encouraged to move her attention away from Max and toward her children in a more productive way. This could be achieved by shifting her into the Earth element along the control cycle. By emphasizing the importance of her stabilizing the family and providing nurturance to Cory, Nora could shift out of the Wood position that was actually promoting Max's excess Fire. Eventually, the two boys and Nora should be moved into a Water position to help cool and control Max's Fire. This could be achieved by utilizing Max's concern and compassion toward his children to generate remorse and temper his Fire.

***Staff Meeting***

Interpersonal relationships are not limited to families, and a number of patterns related to the Law of Five Elements can emerge in organizational structures. At a meeting of a managed-care mental health team, the clinical supervisor was presented with a number of diverse manifestations.

Roger, the team psychiatrist, had finished his training two years previously. While well versed in diagnosis and medical management, he was very insecure about working directly with clients. He became anxious if he had to meet with more than one person, and his ears would turn bright red during the session. At a previous staff meeting, Roger had indicated that he became traumatized whenever he needed to deal with small children. He went to great lengths to ensure that their parents would not bring them in for treatment, preferring to make his diagnoses based on parent description rather than direct observation. If the parents insisted on bringing the children in for the appointment, Roger usually left the session several times to make phone calls or go to the restroom.

> Roger is clearly demonstrating a high level of Water imbalance. His generalized fear and specific anxieties are related to problems in this element. Roger's red ears are indicative of insufficient cooling in the system (ears are related to the Water element), and his frequent trips to the bathroom might be due to the anxiety manifesting in the two Water organs, the Kidney and the Bladder.

Moses, a 35-year-old psychologist, takes things more in stride. In fact, the rest of the staff said that if Moses were any more laid back, he'd be horizontal. Moses had come to the practice after years in a community health agency where he'd had to see a score of patients every week. He was determined not to burn out in his new position. He relished the idea of pondering what to do in each case. Unfortunately, the amount of time he spent in contemplation was triple that he spent in direct service. The rest of the team was being crushed by the load of referrals, while Moses saw an average of only five clients a week. He was very concerned about the rest of the staff, but did not see how he could handle more than his current load.

Moses is demonstrating aspects of the Earth element. His high level of rumination is indicative of the element, as is his concern for other staff members. Moses' lack of movement suggests the presence of damp in Earth, the climatic condition most detrimental to the element.

Nancy, a psychiatric nurse, was the hardest-working member of the team. She happily took on whatever cases she could, and her effervescent personality helped her to handle the pressures of the job. Nancy's problem was that her enthusiasm extended into tracking down the latest approaches to working with clients on an almost daily basis. She was always trying out new therapy techniques that someone had mentioned or she had read about in a journal. Nancy flitted from supervisor to supervisor, always certain that the latest one would give her a fresh approach. As a result, Nancy didn't develop any depth to her therapeutic style and was always struggling to reach successful resolution with her clients.

Nancy demonstrates a number of qualities of the Fire element. Her sense of joy and bright *shen* indicate strong Fire qualities. Her difficulties arise in the inability of one of the Fire organs, the Small Intestine, to fulfill its role of separating the pure from the impure. She constantly assimilates information, but cannot successfully discriminate between what is relevant and what is not. As a result, Nancy struggles to utilize the input in a successful fashion.

Phyllis, a 29-year-old psychologist, had always found it difficult to make it to work. She constantly had colds and sinus headaches, although on some days her absence was due, instead, to her feeling depressed. Since her husband's leaving her, life seemed an uphill battle. She worked hard when she showed up, but that wasn't often. As a result, Phyllis was always overwhelmed by her caseload since she often acquired a lot of clients when she came to work, but then let the cases slide during her absences. Phyllis despaired as to whether she was ever going to feel well enough to get everything sorted out.

Phyllis is primarily demonstrating Metal attributes. Her low energy and depressed affect are related to Metal's function of producing *qi*. The nose and sinus areas are also associated with that element. Phyllis' deficient functioning might have been initiated by the termination of her marriage, her Metal-related grieving precipitating the other symptoms.

There are a number of avenues open to the clinical supervisor for improving the functioning of the team. Figure 14.5 illustrates the designation of staff members. Nancy's difficulties could be addressed by moving her energies toward Earth. She could be asked to choose a single therapeutic style for a period of three months and then to evaluate its impact on her competence and her clients. Moses could also be moved along the promotion cycle by changing his contemplation to action. He could use his skills as a psychologist to design outcome-assessment measures for the team, developing a plan to measure staff productivity and quality. This would utilize Moses' thinking skills, but in a way that would promote action. The statistics generated by his study might also prod him into taking on more active cases. Given the damp nature of Moses' problem, it is recommended that a deadline be established for the implementation of the outcome measures; otherwise, he might ruminate for years on the proper way to design the program.

Phyllis needs to develop the energy to move herself out of her stuck position. This could be done by "feeding" her through the mother element, Earth, encouraging her to develop positive nutritional habits, or to utilize members of her family to generate nourishment on an emotional level. Alternatively, Nancy's joyous Fire could feed Phyllis by

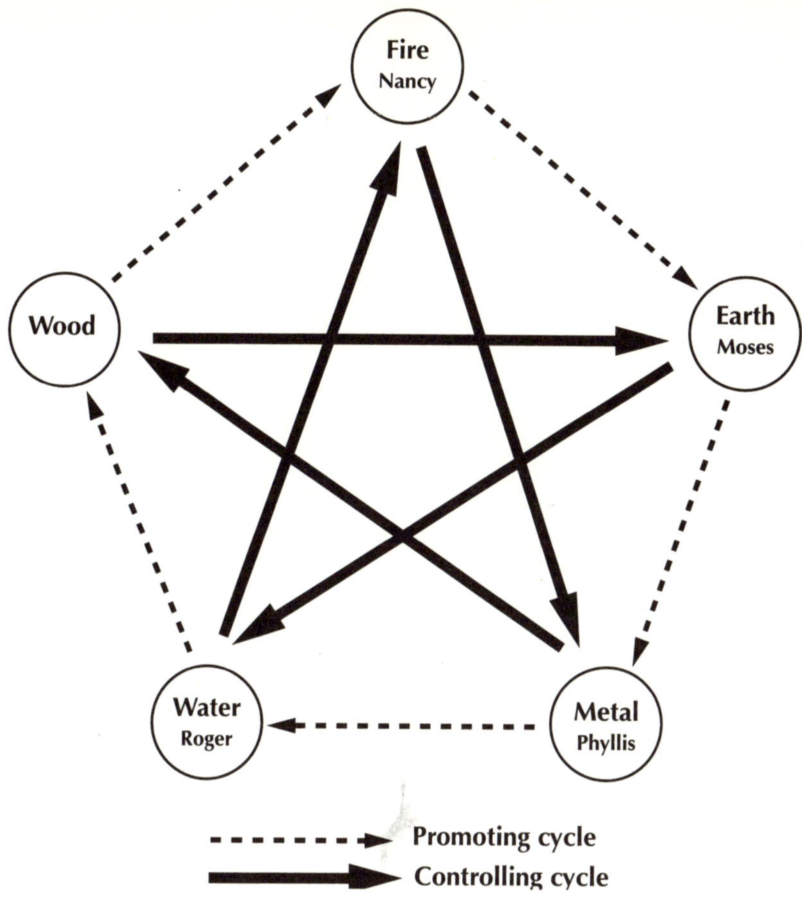


**Figure 14.5.** *Staff meeting.*

infusing her with warmth and compassion for her problems. Phyllis could also be moved toward Wood by using her concern for her clients. She could be encouraged to get angry over how her symptoms and behavior were affecting the well-being of her patients.

Finally, Roger needs to have his fear controlled by increasing rational thought, Earth controlling Water. This could best be achieved by encouraging him to receive sufficient training in how to work directly with clients so that he would feel comfortable with being in the room with them.

■

## In Conclusion

While originally a description of intrapersonal relations, the Law of Five Elements has significant implications for interpersonal systems. By utilizing the promotion and control cycles, a plan of intervention can be established. It is important to realize that, given the interconnection of the elements, input at any point is liable to effect change at another. What is essential is that the flow proceed in a productive direction and not against the system.

## Part Four

# CONCLUDING THOUGHTS

*In the pursuit of learning, every day something is acquired.*
*In the pursuit of Tao, every day something is dropped.*

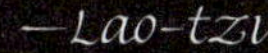
—*Lao-tzu*

Many ideas have been presented and it is hoped that they will sit somewhere in the recesses of the therapist's mind, sending out tiny signals at appropriate times— this is a hot problem, these are Wood attributes, this person has damp characteristics. The intention, however, has not been to make the reader an instant diagnostician in the Eastern sense (for one thing, acupuncturists and herbalists undergo rigorous and lengthy training), but to provide some frameworks for stepping outside typical behavior in the therapist's office. While the details may fascinate, intrigue, and even prove useful, there are several core points that, it is hoped, will travel the distance with you.

**1. Everything is part of the web.**

The human organism cannot be divided into parts that are separate from and independent of each other or the context in which they exist. A systemic approach is inevitable, whether that context is intrapersonal or interpersonal. Climate, culture, family, past history, current events, physiological symptoms, emotional state, the paint on the house next door—everything is woven into the fabric of a person and that person's problem. Depression no more can be a purely psychological problem than it can be a completely physical one. Body, mind, and spirit only exist in relation to one another. Separation creates artificial boundaries that limit effective solutions.

**2. Intent is a valuable tool.**

Practitioners are often sloppy. They don't prepare for sessions, and their focus during appointments can drift and fade. This casualness is a mistake, however, because intent can compensate for the poorest technique or worst choice of intervention. The power of intention may or may not be magic, but it does make a difference. Therapists owe clients their attention—and, for that matter, they owe themselves the ability to focus.

**3. Always seek to strengthen the client's antipathogenic qi.**

Individuals are constantly barraged by stressors; it is an inevitable consequence of living. They cannot insulate themselves from debilitating events, but can only make themselves fit combatants. The concept of antipathogenic *qi* reveals that life can be handled if the organism is strong enough to deal with it. The ultimate goal of therapy should always be to prepare clients to handle their next trauma.

**4. Movement is essential.**

Problems create stagnation and certainty. Thus, a therapeutic objective should be to initiate change in some part of the system. If everything is connected, a stimulus in one sector should result in an impact everywhere else. The choice of where to intervene should be made with care and intent, but a modification at any one point ultimately should affect the whole system. Both the Theory of Eight Principles and the Law of Five Elements suggest appropriate directions for change (movement is better from internal to external or in the direction of the promotion and control cycles). No matter how benign an intervention is, however, clients often become hesitant or fearful when the stability of their patterns begins to change. Therapists must always proceed with the patience and pace that their clients require.

■

**5. Diagnosis should be flexible and serve a function.**

Naming something doesn't solve a problem. Therapists often spend hours deliberating on an assessment, congratulating themselves on the clever diagnosis they have made, and then don't have a clue as to what to do to fix the problem. Psychotherapy can't rely on the Western medical model for solutions, as most of the issues that clients present respond poorly to medical management. For example, although some symptoms of schizophrenia are managed with psychopharmacological interventions, the patient never walks away from medical treatment well and whole. Diagnoses should be working hypotheses, intent transformed into a plan. They are not part of the individual, but an attempt to put past events and current ones into a usable framework. A diagnosis should never be a noun. It is a descriptor that has no solidity, only function. As the individual and the situation change, so should the diagnosis.

**6. Everything is relative.**

The *taiqitu*, the *yin/yang* symbol, clearly demonstrates the relativity of all things. Nothing is absolute. Qualities and problems must always be evaluated by asking: "In relation to what?"A person might be considered anxious in comparison with a placid spouse, but calm in relation to a hysterical parent. By letting go of our absolutes, our truth with a capital "T," we learn both flexibility and compassion.

▪

*People usually fail when they are on the*
*verge of success,*
*So give as much care to the end as to the*
*beginning.*

*—Lao-tzu*

▪

# GLOSSARY

■

**Antipathogenic *qi*:** Energy of the body that operates in a way similar to that of the immune system.

***Jing*:** (j as in English, but with the tip of the tongue on the lower teeth, rhymes with "ring") Essence inherited from our parents. Similar to the genetic code, *jing* is the basis for all growth and development.

***Qi*:** ("chee" as in "cheese") The energy underlying all things; the fundamental substance constituting the universe.

***Shen*:** (rhymes with "when") Vitality and spirit. It is the mold through which essence is expressed.

***Taiqitu:*** ("tye-chee-too") The great polarity, usually known as the *yin/yang* symbol.

***Tao*:** ("dow") The way.

***Xue*:** ("shway") Blood—generally composed of fluids, the nutrients from food, and the energy obtained from breathing.

***Yang*:** (rhymes with "gong") Attributes similar to the sunny side of a slope or of fire.

***Yin*:** (rhymes halfway between the sounds of "sheen" and "shin") Attributes similar to the shady side of a slope or of water.

***Yuan qi*:** ("you-ahn chee") Energy inherited from one's parents. The source of all activity in the body, it can be used, but never replaced.

# REFERENCES

Hou, Z.L. (1979). A study of the histologic structure of acupuncture points and types of fibers conveying needling sensation. *Chinese Medical Journal*, 92, 223.

Lao-tze (1972 edition). *Tao Te Ching:* A New Translation by Gia-Fu Feng and Jane English. New York: Vintage Books.

Madanes, C. (1981). *Strategic Family Therapy*. San Francisco: Jossey-Bass.

Madanes, C. (1984). *Behind the One-Way Mirror: Advances in the Practice of Strategic Therapy*. San Francisco: Jossey-Bass.

Plummer, J.P. (1980). Anatomical findings at acupuncture loci. *American Journal of Chinese Medicine*, 8, 179.

Whiteside, R.G. (1998). *The Art of Using and Losing Control: Adjusting the Therapeutic Stance*. New York: Brunner/Mazel.

*Yellow Emperor's Inner Classic* (Huang Di Nei Jing). Authorship attributed to the legendary emperor Huang Di, and his six physician counselors, who lived circa 2800 B.C. Most likely actually written and compiled between 200 and 100 B.C.

# SUGGESTED READINGS

■

*Chinese Acupuncture and Moxibustion* (1987). Bejing: Foreign Languages Press. A detailed examination of Chinese medical diagnosis and treatment.

East Asian Medical Studies Society (1985). *Fundamentals of Chinese Medicine*. Brookline, MA: Paradigm Publications. A comprehensive overview of Chinese medical diagnostics and treatment. The introduction by Ted Kaptchuk is an enlightening discussion of differences between Eastern and Western approaches.

Flaws, B., & Wolfe, H. (1983). *Prince Wen Hui's Cook: Chinese Dietary Therapy*. Brookline, MA: Paradigm Publications. An interesting look at Chinese diagnostics and treatment through modification of diet.

Hammer, L. (1990). *Dragon Rises, Red Bird Flies: Psychology and Chinese Medicine*. New York: Station Hill Press. A comprehensive look at psychiatry from a Chinese medical perspective. The book offers some interesting insights but is difficult for Western practitioners.

Kaptchuk, T. (1983). *The Web That Has No Weaver*. New York: Congdon & Weed. The best text to acquaint nonacupuncturists with the principles and practice of Eastern medicine.

# INDEX

## E



## F

## G



## H



## I

## J



## K



## L



## M

## N



## O



## P



## Q

## U



## V



## W



## X



## Y